The International Library of Psychology

THE TECHNIQUE OF PSYCHO-ANALYSIS

Founded by C. K. Ogden

The International Library of Psychology

PSYCHOANALYSIS
In 28 Volumes

THE TECHNIQUE OF
PSYCHO-ANALYSIS

DAVID FORSYTH

First published in 1922
by Routledge, Trench, Trubner & Co., Ltd.

Reprinted in 1999
by Routledge
2 Park Square, Milton Park, Abingdon, Oxon, OX14 4RN

Transferred to Digital Printing 2007

Routledge is an imprint of the Taylor & Francis Group

© 1922 David Forsyth

The publishers have made every effort to contact authors/copyright holders
of the works reprinted in the *International Library of Psychology*.
This has not been possible in every case, however, and we would
welcome correspondence from those individuals/companies
we have been unable to trace.

These reprints are taken from original copies of each book. In many cases
the condition of these originals is not perfect. The publisher has gone to
great lengths to ensure the quality of these reprints, but wishes to point
out that certain characteristics of the original copies will, of necessity, be
apparent in reprints thereof.

British Library Cataloguing in Publication Data
A CIP catalogue record for this book
is available from the British Library

The Technique of Psycho-Analysis
ISBN 0415-21088-7
Psychoanalysis: 28 Volumes
ISBN 0415-21132-8
The International Library of Psychology: 204 Volumes
ISBN 0415-19132-7

PREFACE

This little book owes its inception to an address which I gave to the members of the Psycho-neurological Society in London during my presidential year of office, but it includes much more than could be brought forward on that occasion. In its preparation some acquaintance with the subject on the part of the reader has been taken for granted.

DAVID FORSYTH.

INTRODUCTION

I suppose that most medical men who come to practise psycho-analysis have their interest first awakened by reading psycho-analytical literature. They approach the practical side with an adequate or even extensive knowledge of theoretical considerations, but with no greater practical skill than can be acquired by studying the published accounts of analyses made by others. This is at best second-hand observation, and is far from possessing the same value as experience gained by the analysis of even one patient. In point of fact there is every whit as much a technique to be learned here as in, say, operative surgery, and mere reading holds about the same position in each specialty : it is indispensable but it cannot replace practical work. Yet to leave each beginner to work out a technique for himself would mean years of misplaced effort and wasted labour, whereas the hard-won experience of earlier workers in the same field should be his by right of scientific research.

In two ways can this advantage be secured, this service rendered. Either the student gains his practical knowledge by assisting an expert ; in the case of psycho-analysis this implies being analysed—an option the exercise of which I shall consider later. Or he relies on the experience, whether recorded verbally or in print, of those who have already journeyed along the road which he now wishes to follow. And since psycho-analytical technique was first elaborated and written on by Freud, it is his papers we must all take as our guide. Though brief, they are laden with ripe advice and will be utilised freely in the following pages. Standard articles on the same or kindred topics have come from Ferenczi, Abraham, Reik, Stekel, and others. All of these have been published since 1912, but still await translation into English.* In the meantime, many who are taking up analytical work in this country find themselves without any sufficient direction on practical points. Some of them have their work hampered by minor difficulties, whether matters of omission or commission, which they do not recognise or at best do not see how to remove. Others, feeling their own way, stumble into mistakes and fall into technical errors even of the first magnitude.

My present purpose is to try to supply this want. It will be my endeavour to deal from a practical standpoint with analytical precedure, to discuss the various difficulties which are likely to arise, and to show how to meet them and, better still, to forestall them. One qualification at any rate I can claim for this task. When first I took up analytical work ten years ago, none of the papers mentioned above had appeared, and there was no one in this country to turn to for assistance. It was indeed a matter of groping one's way, and there are few possible mistakes in technique which I did not make—except those which my native intelligence saved me from. It is with the still lively recollections of these earlier days in mind that I present the subject to the reader.

It comprises three topics—the analyst himself, the conditions under which the treatment should proceed, and the analysis proper. (1) *The Analyst.*—In the opening chapter will be considered the personality of the analyst and the rôle it plays in the treatment. (2) *The Prerequisites of the Treatment.*—The second chapter will cover the many details and provisions which must be heeded if the analytical work is to go forward in the most favourable circumstances. (3) *The Analysis Proper.*—The largest aspect of the subject is the analytical management of the case. This will be developed in the remaining four chapters.

*Freud's earliest papers appeared in the *Zentralblatt für Psychoanalyse*, Vol. II., Nos. 3, 4 and 9. His subsequent articles, as well as most of those referred to above, will be found in the *Internationale Zeitschrift für Aertzliche Psychoanalyse*, Vols. I., II., III., and V.

THE TECHNIQUE OF PSYCHO-ANALYSIS

CHAPTER I

THE ANALYST

IT is well known that in psycho-therapeutic work the personality of the physician counts for a very great deal. Not only will one physician succeed where another fails, but one and the same physician will number both successes and failures among his cases. Because this is true when no special method of psycho-therapy is followed, and the physician relies on little more than tact and self-confidence, the entire practice of psycho-therapy has undoubtedly and, I think, not unjustly incurred a good deal of obloquy. Disapproval has come, naturally enough, from those who have been trained in scientific method, and see the opportunities for imposition and charlatanry where nothing better is involved than sheer empiricism. Moreover, another serious objection is inherent in this older, haphazard psycho-therapy. It is without any means of ascertaining why its results are good or bad as the case may be ; no matter how extensively it might be employed, it could never lead to the formulation of any rules of practice which would be an assistance on subsequent occasions or enable the technique to be carried some steps nearer perfection.

The same criticism can fairly, it seems to me, be directed against treatment by suggestion. That its results are often brilliant, or, rather, dramatic will be readily allowed, but its failures must be accounted as no less impressive. Yet so far as I can learn no adequate reasons for its success or failure have ever been given. To speak of " good subjects " and " bad subjects " for suggestion leaves the matter where it was. And if, as often happens, the same factor of the personality of the physician is invoked, we are still left with what is little more than a pleasing phrase. Indeed, it seems in the nature of suggestive treatment that it is a bolt shot almost at random, and whether it hit or miss, no one can account for the result in terms precise enough to ensure a better aim next time.

Nevertheless this factor of personality deserves to be examined more closely. It is too widely accepted to be without any significance, and most will agree that certain types of physicians succeed with neurotic patients better, on the whole, than do certain other types. The explanation of this becomes apparent only in connection with psycho-analytical work. Here, as before, personality plays a leading part, and the utility of the method is found to vary with those applying it. Some can attain results which are not to be looked for from others, and every beginner must be prepared to recognise limitations to his capabilities which are set in part by his own personality. But, unlike suggestion, psycho-analysis provides a scientific means of identifying those personal traits which are of help, and those others which stand in the way. It teaches the student how to employ his personality with each patient that comes before him, and enables him in cases which would otherwise be a failure from the outset, to recognise early the causes of the threatened failure, if they lie in himself, and to proceed to their removal one by one. Of no other method of treatment can this be said.

Before making a particular application of of these general statements, we must have clearly in mind the differences in the relation between physician and patient in analytical practice and in ordinary medical practice. This is all the more necessary seeing that most who take up psycho-analysis already have experience of ordinary practice and are therefore liable to carry over into their new work the habits and procedure acquired in their old. Nothing could be more fatal. In ordinary practice the attitude of a physician to his patient includes four aims—first, to take the earliest opportunity of gaining his confidence and establishing a friendly atmosphere ; second, to impress him with his ability to deal successfully with his case ;   third, to give his opinion with due professional authority which may or may not claim *ex cathedra* infallibility ;   and last, to require an implicit obedience in carrying out his advice, he taking all responsibility and the patient relying on his superior, special knowledge.

In analysis the position is quite otherwise. Instead of attempting actively to create a friendly relationship the physician accepts the atmosphere brought by his patient, and towards every change in his feelings—and they will be numberless—adopts a passive attitude ; indeed to proffer friendliness in any way is, with neurotics, likely to invite a rebuff, and in the first encounter it will not be the physician who scores the point. Similarly any scepticism on the part of the patient is not to be taken as inviting any move by the physician to dispel it ; later and at the proper season it will come up to be dealt with in another way. Any claim to professional authority, or still worse to infallibility, finds no place in analytical work ; it would be resented, and in any event could not be maintained throughout the long period of the analysis. While, most dangerous of all, to expect a patient obediently to shelter behind the physician's responsibility would traverse a fundamental principle of analysis which enjoins the exact contrary, namely that the patient must always aim at holding himself responsible, and never lean on the support of the physician.

All this implies that the analyst's first duty is to be passive and not active. He leaves the field to his patient, allowing him complete freedom to reveal his temperament, while he on his part merely listens, follows, notes. In no way and in no sense is he to bid for or show any particular feeling, accept any particular relationship or lead along any particular path. This may sound simple, but is at first far from easy to do. It is difficult for reasons which can be shortly stated. An analysis implies a display of the whole gamut of the patient's moods and feelings. Fear, love, hate, jealousy, obstinacy, mistrust, pride, disgust and all the permutations and combinations of these and other emotions manifest themselves in all degrees of strength, and as we shall learn later are invariably directed at the physician. Love, for example, will lead the patient to try to appeal to his affection ; hate will bring forth anger and all the hard and bitter accusations which it prompts ; obstinacy implies unreasoning opposition to the treatment at every step. Though it is not to be supposed that the analytical thermometer always registers high in respect to these matters, each day comes charged with feeling of some kind, and provided the treatment is running favourably, outbursts of pent-up emotion will occur from time to time.

Now in everyday life any show of feeling on one side brings forth reciprocal feeling on the other—affection stirs affection, anger provokes anger, distrust distrust—but if this were to happen under psycho-analytical conditions the treatment would become impossible and would quickly end. It is for the analyst never to allow his feelings to be played on, although in many, probably in most cases, the patient will try to obtain this ascendency over him. He will do best to train himself to regard every ebullition of emotion merely as a symptom, and just as he would never allow himself to be, let us say, angered by a persistent cough in phthisis or disgusted by hæmatemesis from a gastric ulcer, so these manifestations of feeling pass him by.

But this emotional detachment is more easily written about than achieved. Most beginners would find difficulty in remaining really impassive before even a mild display, let alone a storm of feeling. Some more effective safeguard is needed, and here there would seem to be choice of only three courses.

The analyst may regard himself as a man of great self-control, and think to assure himself that this is security enough.   It may be, but I doubt it.   It would be wiser and truer to see himself as no different from his fellows and as liable as they to be moved by love, annoyance, vanity, timidity.   And in any case to rely on self-control shows that there is something to be controlled, and it is hardly possible for feelings, however checked, not to betray themselves by voice or manner, and probably quite unconsciously.   This course, therefore, is bound to fail because the requisite condition is not that the feelings should be kept in hand, but that they should not be involved at all.

So far as the physician is aware of his emotional susceptibilities, all may go well, but where he is unconscious of them he is on a level with his patient whose cure he nevertheless has undertaken.   If he has done no better for himself, what help can he expect to give his patient ?   In point of fact, psycho-analysis shows over and over again that just so far as he has got the better of his own emotional instabilities (*i.e.*, repressions), so far are his services of value to his patients—

but no farther. Indeed patients are now slow in forming a pretty shrewd estimate of the kind of personality with which they have to deal, and they cannot possibly rely on it where it shows itself untrustworthy. Success as an analyst is, first of all, a case of "Physician cure thyself."

The second and third courses mentioned above are the practical application of this injunction. The student needs analysis himself if he is to do sound work, and here he has choice of alternatives. He may elect to proceed by self-analysis. This possesses the advantage that it can be carried on at times to suit his other work, and that no monetary outlay is involved. Moreover, if he is simultaneously practising analysis on others, he will constantly find, as he listens to the life-histories of his patients, that echoes are awakened from his own childhood. In this way he may hope to piece together a quantity of detail which will enable him to see many of his repressions and release them. Indeed, it may be laid down as a general rule that whenever he finds his own feelings provoked, here is occasion for further self-analysis. But the value of self-analysis is limited, and to other repressions he will remain blind, including some which affect his personality most profoundly.

Yet these would be readily identified by another analyst. The third course, therefore, is to place himself in the position of patient. This is the best course, for in no other way can he be sure of ridding himself of his repressions and all that they imply—partial and biassed views, weaknesses, inconsistencies, some traits in his character stunted, others too dominant. By showing him the worst about himself, and the best, it substitutes tolerance for intolerance and gives a degree of self-knowledge which cannot be gained in any other way. Further, once he is acquainted with the stages of his own psychical development, he knows the psychology of every patient who comes under his care. In a word, he is provided, so far as his natural endowments allow, with a personality in which strength, sympathy, understanding, and love of truth are the main features ; and this is precisely the personality which neurotics must be able to find in any physician who is to be a help to them. Incidentally, the analysis has the additional advantage of teaching the technique.

But it may not be open to all to avail themselves of this preparation, and for some it will be necessary, at first at any rate, to rest content with self-analysis. For these a few remarks may be added on some of the commoner resistances which impede the analysis. This means returning to the subject of the personality of the physician, the rôle of which we can now understand.

It is evident that a good analyst will hardly be made out of a man whose affection or hate is too easily roused, or who is impatient, touchy, suspicious, timid, stubborn, harsh, overbearing or yielding, or who possesses any of many other traits too numerous to specify. But the qualities which are most often overlooked and which come to operate as a frequent obstacle, are those comprised under the heading of narcissism—*i.e.*, vanity, conceit, self-satisfaction, intellectual snobbery *et hoc genus omne*. Narcissism is one of the largest ingredients in the composition of all people, psycho-analysts not excepted,

and may obtrude   itself at many places in
the treatment.   It may lead the analyst to
assume an air of superiority to those seeking
his assistance—a weakness so common among
professional bodies and coteries of all kinds—
and to feel a certain contempt for his neurotic
patients with their never-ending tergiversa-
tions to escape the truth.   But both contempt
and airs of superiority are altogether beside
the point.   More often the subtle play of
narcissism will persuade the analyst to have
in mind the effect of a successful case on his
reputation and the growth of his practice.
There again error is involved, and the consideration (which can only result in making
him over-solicitous for his case—that is, his
own feelings become involved), must be put
aside.   This should not be difficult once
enough experience has been gained to show
how largely the factors of success lie with the
patient himself, and how often he uses every
resource not to part with his neurosis, even
for no better reason than to spite the physician.

    A similar narcissistic bias is responsible for
the common tendency in beginners to assert

a purely technical or theoretical interest in their cases. They may, for example, influence the course of the analytical hour in order to secure conclusions which are of purely theoretical value. Instead of allowing the associations to run freely, as from a dream (in which case the dream may soon be lost sight of), they continually bring the patient back to the starting-point with the object of securing a complete analysis of the dream. The motive here is likely to be either to impress the patient with their skill or to obtain interesting material for publication. In sound analysis both these motives must be renounced. It is undesirable even to study a case in progress from a scientific point of view. Freud emphasizes this when he points out that psycho-analysis provides the twofold opportunity of scientific investigation and of treatment, but is never to be used for the former, scientific ends being reserved until the termination of the case. I read this, however, not as meaning that the analyst is never entitled to practise or experiment on a case, least of all in his early days when he is still learning. Without this help he would find unnecessary difficulty in applying his knowledge and in becoming skilled on the practical side. These grounds, however, show a better motive than narcissism.

But, it may be asked, if on the one hand the analyst does not allow his feelings to intrude, and yet, on the other, avoids the position of a scientific investigator, what attitude remains for him to take up ? The question is of the first importance and can be answered unequivocally once the necessary considerations between patient and physician are kept in mind. The patient is sufficiently handicapped by nervous disabilities to feel the need of extraneous help to restore him to social life ; and for this service he is prepared to pay. The physician, by virtue of his special training and experience, is in a position to render this service, in return for which he charges his fee. The arrangement is mutually advantageous and no obligation rests on either party—the patient is not entitled to claim anything more, even on the ground of having employed this particular physician, nor is the latter given any right to expect gratitude or any special tribute to his skill and ability. The relationship here, as in all professional work, is primarily one of barter and exchange, and this calls for nothing more, but nothing less, from the physician than that he shall at all times do his best, and shall show the customary politeness and consideration of cultured social intercourse. In psychoanalysis, however, these need to be applied under special conditions. Neurotics have difficulty in conforming to this code, and are likely to depart from it even widely ; these occasions must never provoke the physician to follow suit. Again, most neurotics are super-sensitive and quick to seize on any colourable pretext for taking offence ; it is best that these chances should be as few as possible. Lastly, all neurotics are in large measure characterised by views and opinions that are distorted, prejudiced, exaggerated. One result of analytical treatment is to liberate them from these handicaps, but the process can only be gradual, and the physician must never show vexation or even impatience on this account, still less try to force on them views which will shape themselves in due course. Rather let him place himself at their standpoint and provisionally accept their view which, after all, is the only one open to them in their position.

A spirit of tolerance and " sweet reasonableness " is never out of place, though whenever opportunity arises the patient must be brought to recognise his unreasonableness. This, however, should be attempted, not by the physician opposing his view to that of the patient—this would be a crude procedure savouring in analytical work of the brutal— but by waiting until the patient has himself provided all or almost all the evidence needed to open his eyes to the true facts : out of his own mouth he is to be convinced. Even in this the physician must guard against any inclination to score against his patient, or to hurt his feelings for the sake of hurting them. Here a lesson learned at the bedside can be applied with no less advantage. We all trained ourselves, even if we were not taught it, never to hurt a patient when this is unnecessary, but equally never to abstain from hurting if this is in his interests. Similarly in psycho-analysis where our patients' feelings are continually being probed and laid bare, the rule is always to respect their feelings, never hurting unnecessarily; but when the need arises to hurt them—and this occurs in many cases—then to shrink is dereliction of duty. In some cases it is imperative to inflict even a grievous wound—par excellence to a man whose difficulties in life originate in overweening conceit—and nothing less than a mortal blow suffices. But to wound in cruelty or to spare from compassion or timidity—in either case the analyst is at fault.

In conclusion, a few remarks must be added on the relation between physician and patient outside the analysis. This is, in fact, already covered by the rule given above that the personality of the analyst is to be kept altogether apart from the treatment. For this reason it is better that a subject for analysis should have had no social relations with the physician. Not that these need prevent the treatment being undertaken, but they may introduce difficulties, and at the conclusion the pre-existing relations are likely to be permanently changed. But whether the patient is a stranger or not, no social relations

c

of any kind are permissible during the course
of the treatment. At some stages in the
treatment friendly invitations may be expected, but one and all are to be declined on
the simple ground that a fundamental rule
in analysis would be violated. This rule
cannot be too rigidly adhered to, and any
analyst who is rash enough to depart from it
will surely regret it. The same rule should
be applied to receiving presents. Whether
invitations or presents are to be accepted
after the termination of the analysis is another
matter and can be dealt with as may be pre-
ferred. But if the analyst has completed his
task satisfactorily it is improbable that the
question of either will arise, unless it be for a
short time afterwards. In most cases the
patient will soon forget both the analysis
and the analyst, and will feel that no obligation remains to be discharged. In a few
instances only will mutual tastes and interests
supply material for a subsequent friendship,
and in these cases the fact of the pre-existing
analytical relationship is no bar.

CHAPTER II

THE PREREQUISITES OF THE TREATMENT

IN the last chapter it was pointed out that in psycho-analysis the relation of physician to patient is not that which exists in general medicine, and the main differences between the two were discussed. These distinctions are not only to be kept constantly in mind until, by practice, they govern the analyst almost automatically, but they are to be taken into account at every stage and in every detail of the treatment itself. From this it follows that the principles already laid down are to be applied to all the many little points of daily contact between analyst and patient. This is the more necessary because the very fact that the analyst keeps his personality in the background is only likely to provoke the patient's curiosity, and make him seize upon any spare minutes or chance opportunities to satisfy himself as to the kind of individual he

is dealing with. Indeed most patients will
a times make quite determined efforts in
this direction, and will try all manner of
artifices to draw the analyst into the foreground. This curiosity, natural enough in
the circumstances, leads them to seize upon
his every casual remark or action and use it
as the material for a whole series of inferences which may or may not be justified, but
which will assuredly be reflected in their
bearing for days or weeks afterwards. On
the whole, these and other stray influences,
these side-winds blowing fortuitously, impede
rather than expedite the analysis, and it is only
wise to provide against them by giving as
few opportunities as possible for them to
arise. How best to do this will be considered
immediately, but first we must say something
of matters preliminary to the beginning of the
treatment.

The three questions which most patients
will wish answered before deciding on an
analysis are, " How long will it take ? "
" What is the prospect of cure ? " " What is
the cost ? " To deal with these in order. At
the least an analysis takes several months,

and this must be made plain at the outset. Freud gives six to twelve months as the average duration, and it is known that in difficult cases he has found it necessary to continue longer. But the shorter estimate will cover the large majority of cases. I am inclined to add that a student may do well to rest content with cases for a shorter time even than six months,[1] for the reason that he is not likely to be able to go very deep into any case—this can come only with experience—and it may be that the end of three or four months will exhaust his technical resources. Nevertheless his aim should be to penetrate more deeply in each successive case, and in due course he will realise that a year is none too long for a useful analysis.

It seems desirable to give here a warning against the practice of some in accepting cases for so-called " short analysis " when a patient is unwilling or, on account of expense, unable to arrange for more than perhaps a very few weeks' treatment. The objection is twofold. It is not only likely to result in no

---

[1] But see p. 45.

real benefit to the patient, but by leaving him with an erroneous opinion of the value of psycho-analysis, brings the treatment into disrepute. On the other hand, it would be incorrect to assume that so limited a course is never helpful, but the circumstances making this advisable are quite other than those mentioned above. In some cases a short treatment produces good results—even a single interview in which psycho-analytical knowledge is applied, may completely dissipate certain mental worries and depressions and be a turning point in a patient's life—but the selection of suitable cases as well as the conduct of the analysis require some considerable experience. If it is a question of proceeding as it were by short cuts and abridgments, the analyst needs to know his ground well and to be practised in understanding and handling the changing moods of a patient. This comes only after much time spent in the slow and meticulously detailed analysis of several long cases, and a beginner would be well-advised not to attempt any short analysis until he can claim this experience.

The second question—the prospect of a cure—can be answered more shortly. Excluding, of course, cases which, as a rule, are little or not at all suitable for analysis—introverted types such as paranoia, paranoid dementia, and dementia præcox—satisfactory results can fairly be looked for in the extroverted types which figure as cases of hysteria, anxiety-hysteria and phobia ; more difficult and more resistant are cases of obsessional neurosis and those kindred personalities in which stubbornness, narcissism and hate hold sway. In general, the two chief points to be taken into consideration when estimating the probable results of treatment, are age and intelligence. The younger the patient the better, as a rule, is the outlook—I do not doubt that early childhood is the time, par excellence, for rectifying as well as preventing neurotic tendencies—but with adults the years between twenty and thirty are the best, while from middle-age and onwards, less benefit is likely to result. Nevertheless, many men and some women over forty make excellent subjects. In all cases an educated mind counts for much—except when education has meant an uncritical acceptance of what has been taught : the mind in such patients has probably long since lost the faculty of independent observation—but a quick intelligence counts for more. A keen-witted, alert individual, open-minded and perspicacious is a far more hopeful subject than one who has succumbed to authority and tradition.

The third point to be settled before the treatment begins is the question of payment. Whatever the fee, the expense to the patient is likely to be not small on account of the many weeks or months during which it continues. And yet it is not advisable to undertake a case without charging a fee of some kind. It is the experience of analysts, including myself, who have experimented by departing from this rule, that a patient who receives treatment gratuitously does not prove a willing subject, and that an average rate of progress is not to be expected. For one thing he tends to be notably unpunctual and irregular in attendance ; but more serious still, he is almost certain to make no very decided effort to tackle his difficulties as they arise. With a paying patient it is generally an argument of some considerable force, when he is shirking this task and has perhaps declined to speak for the best part of an hour together, to point out that this reluctance on his part implies a pecuniary cost and nothing gained in return. But with a gratuitous case this argument has no cogency, and one of the strongest inducements to go straight ahead is missing.

Even with hospital patients a small sum commensurate with their ability to pay should be required for each attendance. Nevertheless, no matter how small the fee may be, the length of the treatment involves a total expense which puts the remedy out of the reach of many.

In this conection it may be pointed out that, though the cost to each patient is considerable, the earning-capacity of an analyst is strictly limited. Compared with that of any other medical specialist, it is small, and anyone who is looking for a lucrative return for his labours had best employ himself in some other branch of practice. At the most an analyst is not likely to be able to undertake more than six or eight cases at a time, and this necessitates the same number of hours daily of close and continuous application. When, further, it is realised that throughout these hours he is isolated from every other interest—even telephone-calls coming at a critical moment may interrupt and perhaps destroy a psychological situation of first importance to his patient—it will be understood that analytical work makes heavier demands and at a smaller rate of remuneration than any other kind of special medical work.

One further point in the matter of fees. It is undesirable, as it would be inconvenient for payment to be made at each attendance. It is preferable on both sides that accounts should be rendered monthly. This avoids the inconvenience just mentioned, and saves the patient the annoyance of finding that an account of several months has accumulated against him. Not, however, that this arrangement insures him against the reluctance which most of us are apt to feel when called on periodically to part with sums of money. The analyst will sometimes have occasion to notice an interesting manifestation of this. He may find that while the first monthly account is settled promptly and willingly (the patient at that time still appreciating the novelty and prospective easy success of the treatment), the second account (presented when he is deep in mental difficulties, and is discouraged and perhaps resentful of the slow and painful efforts required of him), is paid less readily, and the immediate effects of presenting it are seen in the dreams of the following night, which contain protests against the futility and expense of the treatment.

These three preliminaries to the treatment being settled, the next point is to arrange the times of the attendances. The rule here is a fixed hour for each case. It will not do for the analyst to shift the hour to suit his convenience, if only because his patients will wish to do the same, and this would mean endless difficulty and discontent in adjusting conflicting wants. Speaking generally, male patients find it necessary to ask for the first or last hours of the working day as interfering less with business, while female patients engaged only in household duties have a freer choice. Daily attendance is almost essential for six or at least five days a week. When this is impossible on account of distance or of other claims on a patient's time, an exception may have to be made, but experience shows that to halve the number of attendances per week will more than double the number of months otherwise needed to cover the ground. This part-time attendance also makes it more difficult for the analyst to fit in his cases, and he is likely to find himself unoccupied for one or more hours on some days in the week.

As will be explained later, patients are rarely punctual throughout the treatment, and for days or weeks together may present themselves anything up to half-an-hour or more after their appointment. On these occasions the remainder of the hour is given to them, but no more, the treatment terminating at the end of the allotted time. On the other hand, no matter how unpunctual a patient may be, the physician must allow himself no departure from rigid punctuality. He must always be ready to begin to the minute. And he must close to the minute. Not only is this de-manded in the interests of his subsequent cases, but even if his time is his own it is rarely advisable to run on beyond the hour. To do so is likely to give the impression (and probably a well-founded impression) that he is either specially interested in the patient or unduly anxious about the case ; and either impression is to be avoided. To the student the temptation to depart from this rule of punctual termination may be great because more progress is often made in the concluding fifteen minutes of the hour than in the preceding forty-five, and he may feel reluctant to interrupt when things are at last going so well.

On some occasions the whole hour goes by default, or the patient telephones at the last moment cancelling it on account of not feeling well enough or of having accepted another appointment elsewhere. It will be found that almost all these occasions synchronise with periods of increased resistance to the analysis, and such absences are to be charged as attendances. On a minority of occasions the inability to attend will rest on other grounds such as physical illness or urgent and imperative calls elsewhere ; these, of course, are in a different category.

Even allowing for unexpectedly vacant hours the physician would soon become tired by the close succession of a number of cases and the continuous attention required of him hour after hour, to say nothing of the cramped feeling after sitting so long at work. To obviate this he might allow himself half-an-hour or more of free time now and again, but a better plan is to leave five minutes free every hour—*i.e.*, each patient begins five minutes after the hour, the " hour " really being fifty-five minutes.

From the foregoing it will be apparent that analytical work can only be run with clock-like regularity. But however willing we may be to conform to this, not all patients are as methodical or accustomed to set the same value on time. Most find themselves more communicative towards the end of the hour, and this is naturally the time when they would prefer to remain in conversation. Five, ten, fifteen minutes pass and the next patient's hour is seriously encroached upon. Moreover, this extra time offers one, if not the chief opportunity, to go outside the analysis proper and establish a more personal relationship with the analyst. For these reasons it must be reduced to a minimum. The interval between concluding the analytical work and parting with a patient can be cut down to five or ten seconds if the electric bell summoning the hall-maid is fixed to the wall beside the consulting-room door. At the termination of the hour the analyst passes from his chair to the bell and rings it. Then as the patient rises from the couch, he opens the door and the interview is terminated.

This requires that all hats and wraps should be removed and deposited elsewhere than in the analyst's room. Failing this, there is hardly any limit to the time that may be taken up in donning outdoor wear, and, incidentally, in engaging in conversation. Unless we are prepared to see our day's timetable fall to pieces, we must insist upon this routine.

No difficulty of the kind is likely to arise at the beginning of the hour, except perhaps in the first few days of a case when a patient is inclined by force of habit to open with the small change of everyday conversation. At later stages this disposition usually represents the wish to avoid any analysis on that day. In either case the serious work of the hour is trenched on and valuable time is lost. It is desirable from the outset, therefore, to accustom each patient on entering to pass at once to the couch and to begin his associations forthwith. The physician does not allow himself to offend by opening a channel of conversation ; but after his custmary greeting, he awaits the patient's introductory remarks or actions (and these, be it noted, often bear significantly on what is to follow). Though the physician's attitude is one of reserve and expectancy, he must be quick and responsive in taking up the patient's first moves, and this is all the more necessary when the opening associations are leading to a difficult topic on which a little help and encouragement may be needed.

Yet another kindred point which, though small, is too important to leave unmentioned. Impelled by the same wish to learn what they can about the physician, patients will take such opportunity as arises to exchange views and opinions among themselves. This is one of the side winds already spoken of which disturb the course of an analysis even seriously. Indeed, merely a chance encounter of two patients is enough to send a backwash which will upset the work for days together. In a recent case—that of a young man— progress was suddenly and unexpectedly stopped for more than a week. It then appeared that he had happened to see the patient—also a young man—next on my list each day. His jealousy was instantly roused and, feeling sore against me, he found himself unable to proceed as before. These unfruitful interruptions can be avoided only if patients do not meet. To this end, each one on arriving leaves his outdoor wear in the hall or in a special room ; and then goes to the waiting-room until his time is due. On leaving he passes direct to his hat and thence to the door. In this way the two who are in the house at the same time—one waiting, one leaving—do not meet. Nevertheless, no plan of this sort will work without occasional failures, and if we find an otherwise inexplicable hitch in the course of any case, the explanation should be sought in some such extraneous source. Similar disturbing influences are liable to

D

emanate from relatives and friends with whom the patient may discuss his illness, and it is advisable in every case to give a warning against this, especially as any " leakage," as Freud puts it, of psychical material is prejudicial to the analytical work.

To turn now to another side of our subject. It is customary for the patient to rest throughout the hour at full length on a comfortable couch, with eyes closed and muscles relaxed. Under these conditions, especially if the room is a quiet one, outside distractions are reduced to a minimum, and attention can be given wholly to the thoughts arising from within. The physician's place is behind and close to the head of the couch, beyond the range of view of the patient. By this means he becomes little more than a voice, and the effects of his personal and physical attributes are almost entirely eliminated ; indeed, it is a common complaint by patients that even after months of regular treatment they have only a shadowy idea of his appearance. This, however, is all to the good, and goes far to ensure that impersonal atmosphere which has already been insisted.

By some analysts, on the other hand, this arrangement is held to be superfluous ; with them the patient sits in a chair *vis-à-vis* the analyst, and proceeds very much as in an ordinary conversation. I have made trial of this method in several cases and have finally given it up. Its advantage is that, with the patient always in view, his changes of expression are easier to follow ; but against this is his much greater difficulty in speaking candidly. Add to this that the analyst is himself under the critical eye of his patients for hours at a time, and the balance of choice is altogether in favour of using a couch.

Whether it is necessary to employ pressure of the hand on the patient's forehead, as originally recommended by Freud, in order to force recollections, can be left to the choice of the reader. At one time this was my custom, but it is many years since I abandoned it. Indeed subsidiary details of this kind become of less and less value with increasing experience. Among them might be placed another technical device which too much occupies the time and attention of the student—word-association tests. These, too,

I made extensive trial of at one time, but came to discard except on special occasions, and I have little doubt that any frequent recourse to them indicates a tyro in analysis who has yet to explore the possibilities of the regular technique.

Misdirected energy can also be recognised in another matter which receives too much attention from many beginners—the direct analysis of symptoms. When a patient makes chief complaint of, say, a hysterical symptom, it is not altogether surprising if an inexperienced analyst is persuaded to see it in the same large dimensions, and to feel he should make it the centre of his analytical work. In this he is in some measure approaching the position of treatment by suggestion, which is directed at a symptom without heed to the deeper-lying processes which have produced it. But symptomatic treatment holds much the same place in psycho-therapy as in ordinary therapy—one employs it only for want of a better. It is unscientific in that it treats effects and not causes, and it can add little or nothing to our knowledge of the underlying morbid process ; on the other hand, it often succeeds in relieving symptoms, and is to this extent valuable. True, the analytical treatment of a symptom is free from the reproach of being unscientific, inasmuch as it proceeds from the effect to trace the cause. Nevertheless many beginners, already accustomed in general medicine to place symptomatic treatment in the forefront of their therapeutics, find themselves concentratng on psychical symptoms from little else than force of habit ; whereas the analytical way is from the first to strike deep at the cause, ignoring the effects at any rate for the time being. On these lines symptoms crumble away and disappear without any direct attack, and often a patient is surprised to discover, perhaps weeks later, that he has been relieved.

Another matter on which a beginner is likely to go astray is note-taking. Freud's advice is to take no notes, as the making of them distracts the physician and interrupts the freedom of the associations. As exceptions to this rule he is inclined to recognise written records of dates, fragments of dreams, etc., but even these he defers making until the evening. Not everyone, however, can rely on his memory to this extent, and with most a certain number of notes made at the time will be necessary, but they must be of the fewest. Among them mention may be made of immediate records of *ipsissima verba* of a patient ; these often prove invaluable on the same or a subsequent occasion.

Against the objection to note-taking is the ever-present need of remembering the innumerable details which each case involves. How, then, is this to be done without the written word ? A good deal depends on the kind of attentive attitude with which the patient's life-story is listened to. The analyst may hold himself keenly on the alert with his attention closely focused, constantly saying to himself, " That's important ; I must remember that—and that—and that." This is very fatiguing, and almost always a special point of this kind is forgotten within a day or two, and probably within a few minutes. It is preferable that he should cultivate an alternative attitude, which is the correct one. Without any straining of the attention he gives himself over to a placid, uniform absorption of what is screaming in at his ears, making no effort to remember, still less with any conscious determination to fix this or that detail, but equally allowing no wandering of the thoughts. In this way mental fatigue is reduced to a minimum, even four or five consecutive hours of work leaving only a moderate degree of tiredness behind. Impressions registering themselves in this frame of mind are almost indelible and can be recalled at will. Practice is needed to acquire it, and the student will find that any nervousness or anxiety in himself effectually destroys it. He needs to feel entirely at ease, tranquil and self-possessed.

Perhaps the difference between these two attitudes will be made clearer by a familiar comparison. Listening to a lecturer, some of the audience will be exerting themselves to remember his remarks by categorising and pigeon-holing them under headings and subheadings, and will probably carry away little or nothing in their minds. Others grow more and more interested and are gradually " drawn in " until they lose themselves and pass unnoticed most outside impressions ; on these the lecturer makes a lasting impression.

I might add that in my own case (I do not know whether this is general) analytical details registered as verbal memories may or may not be at my disposal afterwards, but if they are allowed in part at any rate to take the form of visual memories there is never any difficulty in recovering them. It has proved possible when patients call several years after their analysis, to remember the smallest details of their cases—even dreams which they themselves had long since forgotten—and never with any confusion of one case with another. The surprising ease with which this is done—or, rather, does itself—points to an elemental mechanism possessed by everyone, if only it can be made to work.

Yet another question that is sure to suggest itself, even if it is not directly put by the patient. In cases in which the neurosis is intimately connected with some personality in the patient's immediate surroundings—parent, husband, wife, and so on—is removal to another environment desirable during the treatment ? In general, this is not to be recommended. A psychically healthy individual should be able to suffer no harm in such an environment, or, if necessary, to effect the necessary readjustments in himself. One aim of the analysis is to render the patient capable of following either of these courses, and difficulties are not overcome by running away from them. Moreover, by retaining him in the same surroundings continually exposed to the old source of irritation, a condition of nervous tension is kept up which brings out the neurosis to the full, and at the same time provides him with a powerful incentive to persevere with the treatment. But place him under happier conditions, and the neurosis tends to become quiescent (but likely to break out again once this protection is withdrawn), and he will remain satisfied with an analysis which stops half-way. Similarly in cases of phobia, such as agoraphobia, direct exposure to the conditions provoking the phobia will usually facilitate the analysis.

As a last point, reference must be made to the recommendation by Freud as to the treatment of organic disease claiming attention during the analysis. A non-analytical colleague should be asked to undertake this, though simultaneous organic and psychical treatment is inadvisable as a rule, and the less urgent should be postponed. Similarly with cases first coming under observation in which the diagnosis as between psychical and organic disease is an open one, the opinion of a colleague with special experience of the organic disease in question is almost essential.

CHAPTER III

WE come now to the analytical work itself. Here the beginner may again be reminded that technical proficiency comes only with practice, and that this must go hand-in-hand with a study of psycho-analytical literature. Let it be freely admitted that many of the observations he will find in the standard books are not easy to accept at first. Indeed the scientific contributions made by Freud during the past quarter-of-a-century represent nothing less than a revolution in psychology. Is it to be wondered that his discoveries and the theoretical conceptions based on them have been found difficult of acceptance by many who are altogether unfamiliar with the facts he presents, and have grown accustomed to a theoretical psychology of quite another kind ? But to those who are sufficiently inclined to accept his work as to make trial of it in the treatment of psychical disease, my advice would be to accept nothing on a mere *ipse dixit*, though equally to reject nothing, however improbable or disturbing it may seem. Keep an open mind and test, step by step, the validity of Freud's work. To do this, however, implies beginning at the beginning and working steadily forward. There is elementary psycho-analysis, and advanced, and not all critics of the latter have put themselves to the trouble of mastering the former. Yet the simple should precede the complex. Begin, therefore, with practical observations on patients (and on yourself), and seek to establish in them the elementary facts already discovered by Freud and his followers. Gradually enough material will be collected to enable you to begin to test the theoretical structure of psycho-analysis.

Inasmuch as any one case is not likely to illustrate in itself more than a fraction of the whole subject, and each new case is sure to present features not previously encountered, it might be preferable to begin on several cases simultaneously, perhaps changing them after a few weeks for others. This would seem all the more desirable since no analysis by a beginner goes very deep, and by taking up more cases than one he would have a wider field of investigation. Nevertheless, I would recommend the alternative course—to concentrate time and energy on one case over a long period. For one thing, the aim in analytical work is not the easier one of exploring widely over horizontal levels, but the much more difficult one of penetrating vertically to deeper layers, and how to do this can best be learnt by something in the nature of an intensive study of one case. Simultaneously, if you wish, and time allows, carry on more superficially with two or three other cases, but it is only by working hard at the first case that you will discover the real problems of analysis and learn how to meet them.

Then, again, by no means every case is suitable for a beginner who needs to be circumspect in making his choice. He must leave alone for the present introverted characters, obsessional cases, obstinate, sadistic and negative types (*i.e.*, all with pronounced anal-erotic characters) ; narcissistic types are often troublesome. He would do best to select an extroverted type, one with anxiety-symptoms and especially a case of anxiety-hysteria. The desiderata in respect of age and other particulars have already been specified on p. 23.

One word more by way of preliminary. In the following account, in which it is assumed that the reader is familiar with what is meant by "free association," nothing will be said about the technique of dream-analysis. Not only is this too big a subject for discussion here, but it has been completely dealt with by Freud in his "Interpretation of Dreams," and without a close study of this work no one is in a position to undertake analytical treatment.

Once the analysis has been decided upon, the sooner a beginning is made the better. Delay gives an opportunity for that play of emotions around the physician which is known as the "transference." This will be fully discussed in the next chapter, but for the moment it may be explained that in every case the patient receives an emotional impression of one kind or other of the analyst, and that this is likely to deepen day by day until it soon has taken firm hold. Only if the treatment begins at once can this development be kept under observation and dealt with appropriately. Left to grow unwatched by the analyst and, in all probability, unrecognised by the patient, it will surely become an effective bar, and may require much time and labour to come up with and remove.

Arrange, therefore, to take up each case at the earliest possible moment. Begin, if you like, with a preliminary explanation of the nature of the treatment, but make this brief. Some account of free association, of dreams and fantasies, and of the decisive importance of childhood as the key to adult character will probably cover all that need be explained at this early stage. Theoretical or purely technical points have no place at present. In so far as it is necessary for the patient to become familiar with them, there will be ample time in the months ahead to put him in possession of all that matters; though even then, guard against the common fallacy that because both these aspects are throughout of leading importance to the physician, there-

fore they have a special interest to the patient.
An analysis, remember, is not primarily a
scientific inquiry : it is an emotional experience (conducted, it is true, on scientific
lines), and emotions dry up at the mere
glimpse of scalpel or microscope.

No better opening can be made than,
accepting the suggestion of Freud, to invite
the patient to tell you everything about himself. You cannot at present know very much
about him, and you want to know. Let him
therefore tell everything that comes to his
mind, and as it comes to his mind. Perfect
candour will best help him and you. Meanwhile, your own rôle will be little more than
that of a listener.

In this way the patient is accustomed from
the first to complete freedom in choosing his
starting-point, no leading questions are put,
and indeed no questions are put at all except
by way of elucidation of the narrative.
Should he ask, as often happens at first,
where to begin or what to pass to next, let
him know that the choice is his. Least of
all is he to attempt any systematic presenta-
tion of his life-history, but always to tell it

just as it comes to his mind. Whence it follows that the story is given without any consecutiveness, chronological or categorical, and herein lies one of the first tests of the analyst. Among this mass of tangled detail, much of which is of little value, lie scattered the significant facts bearing on the case. It is for him to recognise them, collate them, and store them in his memory for future use. This is all the more necessary, as few patients can readily forgive the analyst who shows he has forgotten any particular entrusted to him even weeks before—a particular, perhaps of no great intrinsic worth, but costing something to communicate and therefore liable to provoke a sense of disappointment and hurt should it come to be forgotten.

It is important to note that this freedom in the matter of mental association lends itself to exploitation, and may easily be used by a patient to defend himself against any serious work. This usually happens at times when a topic is looming ahead which he wishes to avoid. He then talks readily but superficially, and at the end of the hour has uncovered little or nothing of any consequence.

E

When his attention is drawn to this, as it must be, the almost certain reply is that he has indeed strictly obeyed his instructions to say everything as it rose in his mind; nothing else has come, and he infers that the blame rests with the method and not at all with him. Discursive associations of this nature are of almost daily occurrence in one case or other, and may waste a good deal of time; they figure, therefore, as a leading difficulty in the work. How to deal with them will be discussed later (Chap. V.), but for the present it must be made clear that they are not necessarily valueless. Even when they keep entirely on the surface it may be possible to detect a deeply-hidden thread running through them all, so that the apparently casually uttered thoughts serve only to disclose the personal topic which they are intended to mask. The need of recognising this hidden material will justify us in giving space to an example.

Throughout a great part of one sitting, the patient—a family man—after mentioning that he had no dream to recount, spoke of nothing but the attractions of travel in the East.

The warm climate, bright colours, lavish vegetation and primitive customs were all set out in contrast with this chill and cheerless England of ours. He spoke of the " call of the East," quoted from books on oriental travel, and described a recent exhibition of paintings of Indian life. For the time being his predominant wish was evidently to get away from England and tour the East.

He had never before expressed this dissatisfaction with his own country, but there could be no doubt of its strength this particular morning. True, he had mentioned previously that as a young man he had first quitted the parental roof in order to visit the East ; one of his reasons at the time was to get away from his mother who had begun to jar his nerves, and another was to learn something of oriental types of beauty. The recollection of this earlier episode in his history suggested to me that some similar motives were probably responsible for the unexpected revival of his *Wanderlust.* So, after listening a while, I asked had he had occasion within the past twenty-four hours to be annoyed or disappointed with his wife ? Thereupon he opened a topic which he said he had many times wanted to speak about, namely, his relations with his wife—how she was cold and unresponsive, while he was ardent—and the outside temptations to which these exposed him and against which he had continually to fight.   Only the previous night, after a lapse of several months, he had suggested going to her room, but she refused on the score of being tired, and this led to an open quarrel, each maintaining an opposite view.

To complete the analytical interest of the incident he now remembered that he had had a dream after all.   He was out walking with his wife on his arm, but they had difficulty in keeping step.   Then he found himself handing her to a passer-by, while a lady of his acquaintance came forward and slipped her arm in his.

In this case the associations which at first seemed trivial and entirely superficial became significant when they were seen to circle round this one topic.   They gave expression, very allusively but none the less surely, to his disappointment, and so led direct to a principal cause of his anxiety-symptoms.

Apart from superficial associations, another not dissimilar difficulty arises when a patient prepares his story beforehand each day. He may explain and indeed believe that this is to expedite the analysis. Its effect, however, is the reverse, because it usually implies extensive censoring, and in any case is contrary to the rule that the associations are to be taken just as they come during the hour. Indeed, it is preferable that a patient should not spend time introspectively in this way, or give two thoughts to the analysis during the rest of the day. An exception to this must be made where he is anxious to complete some memories recently dealt with; but here the intention is plainly to help.

Yet again, much time can be unprofitably spent in too copious a narration of actual (*i.e.*, current) experiences. These have their value, especially in the later stages of the treatment when the patient's day-by-day behaviour under varying conditions is being correlated with the findings of the analysis, but for the most part they involve only surface reactions, and are little calculated to uncover any deeper tendencies.

With increasing experience it becomes not difficult to piece together the significant fragments of the patient's broken story. Gradually, and even within the first week or two, the material coming to hand should enable at any rate the leading complexes and fixations to be identified (especially parental and other family attachments), and it may even be possible to postulate events and experiences which have not been mentioned and are as yet entirely forgotten.[1]   Other complexes, however, come up only after a lengthy analysis—for example, the very important castration-complex, whether in men or women, is usually one of the last to appear, and a beginner must not be surprised if it eludes him altogether in his earlier cases.

Now let us look for a moment at a rather more advanced state of the analysis.   Prac-

---

[1] It is here that criticism has been levelled against the analytical method in that it reads this or that into a patient's life-history on what is supposed to be the slenderest foundations, and will even maintain facts which the patient is not aware of and would stoutly deny.   Nevertheless, conclusions of this kind can be safely drawn.   I am never able to see in this anything more remarkable or improbable than are the inferences of, let us say, a game-hunter on finding a single spoor or a branch broken or cropped.   The same niceness and reliability of inference is found everywhere in general medicine, where it is a matter of trained observation supported by the united experience of many

tically all the more readily accessible struc-
tures—fixations and complexes—represent reactions to the outer world. They tell of
external influences upon the patient, and show
the train of consequences flowing from each.
But in all such there is another factor involved, apart from anything in the outer
world. This is the character of the individual
exposed to the influence. It is obvious that
identical experiences will affect different
natures diversely at the time and afterwards.
Take, for example, two children each sub-
jected at the same age to the same psychical
trauma—say, the death of the mother. Both
may well be left with a powerful mother-
fixation, but nevertheless the effects in the
two cases will certainly not be identical and
will almost certainly be dissimilar in many
respects. This is to be accounted for by
differences in character.[1]

Behind and beneath complexes and fixations
we recognise characters, and an analysis is

[1] A special use of the word " character " in psycho-analysis
needs mention. Ordinarily it implies the sum of qualities in
any person, but psycho-analytically we speak of this as his
" characters "—i.e., character, in this special use, is rather the
equivalent of " trait of character." It is in this sense that it
will from now be used in the following pages.

never to be accounted complete until these have been uncovered ; they are the buried foundations upon which the building has taken shape. This, however, is work for more experienced hands. It is concerned not only with more obvious distinctions, such as between extroversion and introversion or even between hetero-erotism and homo-erotism, but with the fundamental partial tendencies of exhibitionism and observationism, sadism and masochism, with narcissism and auto-erotism including anal, urethral, oral and respiratory erotism. Only as these are brought into definition—and this may well mean a long analysis—will the strongest un-conscious tendencies as well as many trivial peculiarities in a patient be understood. Strange to relate, it will then be found that a great deal in the behaviour of each patient is directly a repetition of his infantile be-haviour under the stimulus of the various erogenous zones, especially the oral and anal zones. Nevertheless, though this deeper analysis is advanced work, the beginner should find it an assistance to have this twofold division set clearly before him. First and more obvious, the complexes and fixations ; these are chance accretions, products of environmental conditions. Second and fundamental, the characters which are innate (? hereditary). The two together make up the personality, but it is the characters which determine the form of the super-structure.

In approaching this more difficult work the student should remember that we have three sources from which to learn the characters of any patient. These are (1) memories, especially infantile memories, (2) dreams, and (3) the transference. The transference will be dealt with at length later on, but a few words about the others must be given. Inasmuch as the main lines of character are traced for all time within a very few years of birth, and since it is in early childhood that they are simplest and most easily recognised, the value of infantile memories is evident. Over and over again it will be found that a single memory from this period, provided it includes the manner in which the child reacted to the occasion, throws a flood of light on this question. Dreams owe their value in the same connection partly to the freedom with which they express all tendencies, partly to the symbolism which, almost at a stride, carries the present back to the infantile past, and partly to the fact that in the later stages of an analysis, after the resistances have been mostly overcome, dreams often deal in the most outspoken and almost uncensored fashion with the original primitive impulses.

To return now from this digression to the earlier stages of the analysis. Although we may expect and indeed need to see more deeply into our patient's psychology than he can himself, it would be the mark of a very clumsy beginner to endeavour to convey to him forthwith what we have discovered. Yet this mistake, which is a serious one, is all too often made. It may be many weeks before he gains sufficient insight as even dimly to recognise what is already patent to his analyst. To attempt to force this upon him will not only fail, since his view is from another standpoint, but is likely to be resented as unfair and biased; and we have difficulties enough to contend with in every case without provoking more by want of everyday tact.

Even if he accepts or, rather, acquiesces in what we might try to get him to see, the psychical effect is quite other than when the recognition comes from within; and it is this latter alone which has therapeutic value.

But it may be objected, this leaving him to go his own tardy course is surely a waste of time. Is there nothing that will quicken his steps ? Let it be remembered that psychical changes, modifications in temperament, transitions from the neurotic to the healthy, come but slowly and in due succession. Even those cases are no exception in which extensive changes seem to come about overnight, as it were. In these the material has been gradually prepared until only a touch was needed to bring the laborious work to the surface. Moreover, slow changes are preferable, because more enduring, whereas a lightly-won success may prove only transient. All through the months of the analysis this process is going on, and more is not to be looked for. Remembering this, then, we can answer our question in this way. For some time ahead we can watch our patient step by step nearing the recognition which we are waiting for him to make. We see him one day approaching, the next withdrawing, as his feelings sway him ; but, on the whole, he comes nearer. When at last he is almost, but not quite, able to see the thing for himself, then is the time to interpose. Present him with all the collated facts he has given, and so force to a decisive issue the conviction which has been slowly shaping itself.

Just how this final show of force is to be made—whether the steel fist should be gloved in velvet or used naked—must depend on the type of the case before us, but whichever the choice, do not forget that it is a steel fist you have elected to use. With some temperaments it is best to force them gently from the position they are almost prepared to relinquish to the other which is now ready for them (" May it not be that——? " " It looks as if——? ", and so on) but with others violence, short and sharp, is necessary, and the facts must be driven home with every ounce of energy. No harm is done thereby, for once the position is evacuated as untenable, the patient cannot understand why he clung to it so tenaciously, or resent the efforts that helped him out.

The mention of force brings us to a question which has been receiving a good deal of attention lately, namely, whether active interference by the analyst is permissible. In the technique hitherto an emphatic negative to this has been accepted. From the earliest days Freud emphasised the need of an entirely passive rôle by the analyst, who is to leave the patient to work out his own salvation, as it were. It is on these lines that his followers have worked, the disadvantage of slowness of therapeutic results being outweighed, it was held, by their spontaneity in respect of the patient. But the whole question was raised quite recently when Freud recorded the good effects in agoraphobia of exposure to the conditions which would precipitate an acute anxiety attack.[1] Some years before this, however, a remarkable case of hysteria was published by Binswanger, in which his very active interference was altogether beneficial.[2] Last year at the Inter-

[1] *Zeitschrift*, vol. V., p. 61.
[2] *Jahrbuch für Psychoanalitishe und Psychopathologishe Forschungen*, III., 1.

national Psycho-Analytical Congress, Ferenczi read a paper reviewing the question and supporting the new development.[1] Other opinions are likely to be available in the near future. My own experience is that in most cases moments come when this force can be applied effectively, beneficially and with an economising of time, while on other occasions in the same cases it would be unavailing. There are "psychological moments" in analytical work as in everyday life, when things can be brought about which at other times are impossible. They are not difficult to recognise, and good and not harm comes from turning them to account.

[1] *Weiterer Ausbau der aktiven psycho-analytischen Technik.*

CHAPTER IV

THE reader will recall that in an earlier chapter mention was made of the transference which at a first glance was described as the play of a patient's emotions about the personality of the physician. It is now time to deal with the subject at length. This importance is due to it for three reasons especially—it is a feature of every analysis, it counts more than anything else in facilitating or impeding the work, and on it directly depend the therapeutic results. It is the only healing power with which the physician is invested, and yet, as Freud emphasises, it provides the hardest situation for him to handle. The student, therefore, needs to obtain a clear appreciation of its nature, its forms, and the rôle it plays in the treatment.

In a word, transference is the feelings, the emotional attitude, of the patient towards the physician. Though it has been studied only in connection with psycho-analysis, it is found everywhere in daily life. Suppose two persons, A and B, meeting for the first time : each at once likes or dislikes the other. No matter whether they know anything or nothing about each other, an emotional attitude of some kind is assumed even within the first moment or two. It may or may not be within their power to account for it, and often when it is not—when it is " instinctive," as people say—it goes all the deeper and is more lasting. This is an everyday example of transference. A special example may be seen between a patient and his (non-analytical) doctor. The patient has confidence in him and feels fully content to entrust himself and his case to his hands ; though with another doctor this trust may be impossible, or becomes undermined and disappears. How much this transference counts for in ordinary medical practice every doctor knows, but in psycho-analysis where it is a matter of the patient disclosing every intimate detail of his life—details which have hitherto been guarded as secrets from everyone—its importance is a hundredfold. And just as in ordinary practice this reliance may grow into a dependence which is little helpful in a professional relationship, the same development under analytical conditions would raise almost insuperable difficulties in the way of further treatment.

How, then, in the first place are we to account for the transference ? Given an impression received from without, we are all disposed to respond by a stirring of feeling of whatever kind. Whether the impression is of colour, sound or form, or, in the case of other persons, of physique, voice and so on, these provoke an emotional response, varying in kind and degree, which is the feelings we entertain towards the source of the impression. But the nature and intensity of these feelings are determined by previous occasions when the same or a similar impression was received ; we hear someone expressing certain views, and we like him because we are already partial to those views. But more often than some care to acknowledge, we are primarily influenced by physical impressions, and only those who have educated themselves to require more

F

than this are chiefly responsive to impressions
of another's character as revealed by behaviour and opinions. Yet here again it is a
matter of extending to the new acquaintance
the same feelings of like or dislike which we
have previously associated with the traits we
recognise in him. A and B, when they meet,
bring with them all their earlier emotional
prejudices, and each responds to the other
accordingly. Each *transfers* to the other the
feelings which have been stirred in similar
situations perhaps many times before. Yet
only rarely will anyone be found to posess
enough knowledge of himself to identify the
particular attributes in the other which
provoke the feeling, still less to trace the
earlier occasions for it, and, least of all, to
recall the first and most significant occasion
of all. Yet nothing less than a knowledge of
all this is required if he wishes to understand
his emotional idiosyncrasies.

In not many cases, however, is this transference of so simple and uncomplicated a kind.
Rather will different traits rouse conflicting
feelings of unequal intensity ; but on the
whole the balance will be for or against. If

the acquaintance is continued, the balance may fluctuate from this side to that, and for a time dislike on the whole will alternate with liking on the whole.

Under this condition of continued association a fresh complication may arise. Should A at any time find himself, let us say, opposed to B, his feelings and behaviour will be influenced thereby, and he will react to this opposition precisely as he did on a previous similar occasion when he encountered opposition. The generalisation from this is equally true, and it may be said that each psychical situation that develops will affect each of them in the way it has customarily affected him in the past.

Now let us see how this helps us to understand the question of transference. Each patient who comes for treatment brings with him a temperament which has been shaped and moulded by countless emotional experiences, by far the most effective of which are impressions received in childhood. He possesses all the emotions with which human nature is endowed, and has come to attach them in varying kind and degree to everything in his outer world, according to the circumstances of his upbringing. By force of oft-repeated habit he has his own temperamental way of reacting to each and every psychical situation. Incredible though it might seem to him, his feelings and behaviour under any given circumstances are already determined by his psychical past. Now during the course of the analysis each and all of these situations will be repeated either in the actual setting of current circumstances or by reviving the memories of earlier situations. In either case the same old emotions are roused and *transferred by him to the analyst*, just as though it was the analyst who was primarily and solely responsible for stirring them.

As seen by the analyst in his first case or two, this continuous but changing transference appears as a succession of emotional states, probably very difficult to understand. To-day the patient will twist the analyst's words out of their meaning, impugn his motives and heap blame upon him which seems altogether undeserved. To-morrow— nay, even a few minutes later—he will be hanging on his words, expressing open admiration of his skill and gratitude for his assistance. With rather more experience the analyst discovers that these waves of emotion are directly related to the subject that is being dealt with at the time. They depend little or nothing on himself, if only because he does not change from hateful to lovable day by day, but are the emotions stirred in the patient by each day's work. They are revived from earlier experiences to be transferred to him.

By the full recognition of the fact that it is not he who is responsible for the transference, that it is neither a reflection on him nor any compliment to him, but that it is derived from others who have previously played a leading part in his patient's life, by recognising this the physician has gone a long way towards eliminating any reciprocal response (countertransference) in his own feelings—of meeting anger by anger, or love by love. Both pass him by, and he is content merely to watch and study the features of the case before him.

To go one step further. Any emotion which has been repressed and pent up at some previous time may appear in the transference.

This leads us to an important discovery which can be tested in every patient. Such emotions have remained attached to bygone memories, but once they appear in the transference they are thereby permanently severed from their out-of-date (and probably useless) attachments, which then lose their emotional value. Simultaneously the emotional significance of the physician is enhanced, and this is the situation which calls for careful handling. How to deal with it is a matter that will be taken up immediately ; suffice it to say that this new attachment to the analyst is both desirable and necessary, but only as a temporary expedient, as a half-way house to something preferable.

As might be supposed, the emotions brought to the surface by the analytical work are not always exhibited in the same degree by different patients. Some show them openly and without restraint, but others try hard to hide them ; and the latter are by far the more numerous, since neurotics as a class have schooled themselves to suppress their feelings and are often ashamed to give them even a moderately free rein. Nevertheless this

" abreation," or actual experience of repressed
emotion is one of the most useful conditions
of successful analysis, and every encouragement is to be given in " working off " the
accumulated nervous energy ; subject always
to the one condition that it shall find outlet in
words only, and never in actions. Patients
again vary widely in the intensity of the
abreation that is needed to produce therapeutic results, and while some are from time to
time overwhelmed by their feelings, others
come through as successfully without ex-
periencing more than agitation. But with
most, as the original infantile sources of these
feelings are broached, a flood of emotion
rushes forth, and the analyst will become
familiar with incidents in which, for example,
a patient is given over to the intensest jealousy
of a relative who stood in his path in his
nursery-days, or weeps for hours in recalling
the death-bed scenes of a hitherto forgotten
parent.

A few pages back the transference was
named as one of the three sources of information regarding characters. How it serves
this purpose will now be apparent. The lead-

ing emotional traits of each patient determine
the leading features of the transference, so
that love, hate, fear, mistrust and so on appear
in the transference in much the same proportions that they fill in his nature.   Both love
and hate, of course, are present in all, but in
very different proportions, from much love
and little hate, to much hate and little love.
Of all types those with much hate are the
most difficult analytically, especially as this
is usually associated with strongly developed
sadism and much obstinacy.   These consti-
tute the anal-erotic characters ; they are to
be found in all cases of obsessional neurosis
(it is on this account that they are difficult
to analyse), and are responsible for introverted
types, especially those with paraphrenic
features (which are not analysable except in
the milder forms in children).   On the other
hand, extroverted types with their essentially
affectionate dispositions lend themselves best
to analysis.

We are now in a position to define more precisely the attitude that may be expected at
the outset from any patient.   The transference becomes a matter of his earlier emotional

life, in other words, of those persons who played the leading rôles in his life. But with almost all of us this pre-eminence is to be attributed to the parents of our childhood. Every patient, therefore, takes up towards the analyst (if he is a man) the position he came in his childhood to assume towards his father (towards his mother, if the analyst is a woman). According as he liked his father, disliked him, rebelled against him, feared him, mistrusted him, so will he behave towards the analyst. How faithfully this early association is reproduced, even in its finest details, can hardly be credited until it has been witnessed. And just as this is the key to understanding a great part of the patient's transference, so does his behaviour to the physician reveal by reflection the parent of his childhood.

As a corollary to the above it follows that our first interview with a patient is of decisive importance. It is the occasion of the first linking-up of the physician's personality with the patient's psychical past, and the impression then received will not easily be changed ; for though he may be neither observant nor educated, his unconscious mind cannot but register some kind of record or the physician's personality, disclosed, it may be, equally unconsciously. It is advisable, therefore, to arrange this first interview only when ample time is available, since no neurotic patient likes to be hurried away with only half his story told. As a beginner it may be enough if you do nothing more at this interview than abstain from arousing any active opposition ; a sympathetic hearing of his story will usually ensure this much. But with more experience you will be able to combine this with a more active and penetrating investigation. By occasional questions—here to draw the patient out more fully, there to direct his thoughts along another channel—you will be able to test his emotional reactions in many directions, and touching lightly with your probe, to recognise the complexes and many of the details of the case before you. It need hardly be said that the slightest of touches must be used, and that from first to last no hurt must be inflicted. Least of all should any attempt be made to criticise, or to draw attention to the errors, inconsistencies and biases which are likely to appear. The present purpose is to allow him to disclose himself, and to recognise his points of view, accepting them *in toto* as the necessary and only possible starting-point of the analsyis. Again, almost every patient has his special desiderata as regards his physician—if not that he possess this trait, then that he lack that—and will tacitly and inferentially show his desire for information on the point. These questions may be answered, also tacitly and inferentially, and in general any preliminary doubts with regard to the nature of the treatment cleared out of the way. Now and again patients will present themselves half-expecting to find you a monster of iniquity, " sex-mad," and with every vice written large on your countenance. These are they who have had psycho-analysis represented to them by the heated imagination of some of its opponents, and as it speaks much for their courage and clear vision that they should nevertheless have decided to undergo the treatment, it is only due to them to let them know you for what you are.

Passing now from the preliminary interview to the subsequent course of the transference,

we must recognise that though there is no
feeling or shade of feeling which may not be
utilised for transference, all can be reduced to
two forms—positive transference (= love)
and negative transference (= hate). Some
practical considerations special to each of
these must next be dealt with.[1]

THE POSITIVE TRANSFERENCE.

The positive transference ranges from mere
friendliness to falling violently in love. Maintained at a mild degree, it provides the best
atmosphere in which to carry on the work, it
expedites the analysis by keeping many emotional obstacles out of the path, and conduces
most surely to a successful ending. It is
described by Freud as the bridge by which
the patient can be led from illness to life.
For this purpose it should be allowed to
remain at a moderate level. If, as happens
not infrequently, it rises higher or is replaced
by a negative phase, it should be restored as
soon as possible. Day by day watch is to be
kept on its variations, information being
obtained, apart from the ordinary manifesta-

[1] The word " transference," when not qualified by " positive "
or " negative," is customarily used to denote the positive form.

tions of feeling which most can recognise, from two sources—the patient's attitude towards the analysis and its circumstances, and from his dreams.

One of the most constant signs of a positive transference is punctuality in keeping the daily appointment ; while during periods when the transference increases, patients may present themselves a quarter-of-an-hour or more before time. Simultaneously they begin to express admiration, not indeed directly of the physician, but of his furniture, fine pictures and so on, commend the civility of his hall-maid, and inquire about his family. They grow careful about their appearance, and show the range of their ties and dresses. All this time they co-operate in the analysis to the best of their ability. But should the transference begin to get out of hand, the work is retarded, and little or no progress may be made for days or possibly weeks together. Thoughts cease flowing, the mind becomes blank and long pauses of silence fill the hour. In some cases in which an intense shyness shows itself, the patient becomes mute and unable even to answer when spoken to.

It is in the dreams, however, that the first and surest evidence of the transference and its changes is to be found. In most dreams brought for analysis, the physician figures somewhere, and it is not difficult to recognise from the way he is dealt with, the thoughts and feelings that are being entertained for him at the moment. He may be represented outspokenly as himself, but often his personality is disguised as a previous doctor who has treated and been liked by the patient (not uncommonly a long-forgotten doctor from nursery days is evoked for this purpose). On many occasions he appears as a priest, a father, a policeman, or as a fine animal such as a lion or a horse. In the dreams of medical men undergoing analysis he is not infrequently depicted as an ophthalmic surgeon ; the unconscious mind, with its curious facility for punning, representing him as an I-surgeon.

Whatever the disguise adopted in the dream, the nature and state of the transference can be readily tested in two ways. First, from the surroundings of the analyst in the dream itself. In one dream, for example, he was a lion walking with the patient in a sunlit flower-garden; the situation here being altogether agreeable, the positive nature of the transference is obvious. But still more information can be obtained from the associations to the thought of the figure representing the analyst. In another dream a policeman was knocking at the door, notebook in hand, to make inquiries, but the patient hesitated to let him in. Here the thought of the policeman suggested strength and patience, authority and order—all positive indications; but the transference was not quite so simple because the hesitation revealed both resentment and fear with reference to the analyst.

Just as the positive transference is the only authority conceded to the analyst, so it is the measure of the willingness of the patient to obey the instructions given to him. It is largely for this reason that a moderate degree is so helpful. It induces the patient to conform to the conditions of the treatment, and fortifies him in carrying through what is nothing less than an arduous and painful task. The physician on his part is to utilise it for both these ends, but for none other. It is true that transference alone can remove symptoms at any rate for a time (and this is probably the explanation of successful treatment by suggestion, and of cures at holy places), but Freud warns against using it for any such purpose. This, he points out, is not psycho-analysis ; this method on the contrary employs the transference only as a means of overcoming the patient's resistance— a fundamentally important distinction.

One or two obligations of a less important kind are cast on the physician in connection with the positive transference. In the first place, it becomes necessary to revise a rule which was laid down in an earlier chapter. It was stated that the analyst must keep his feelings outside the treatment altogether. This has now to be qualified in one respect. It often happens that a patient in whom the transference is positive but in no way excessive will declare his complete inability to face any further analysis without an explicit assurance of the sympathy and continued esteem of his physician. Needless to say, this difficulty should never be allowed to remain. Further, it is in many cases helpful rather than the reverse for the analyst to communicate to his patient something of his own life—he who seeks confidences, says Freud, must be ready to give them. Without this the impersonal character of the analyst, known by little more than his voice, gradually becomes a provocation to the patient, who not unnaturally feels the need of being satisfied that, after all, he is dealing with someone of flesh and blood like himself. In this connection it might be added that most patients find it helpful to learn of cases with similar details to their own. Such help, however, is not to be given in order to lessen their difficulty in overcoming a resistance.[1] This they must do unaided, and only after they have battled with it successfully should the information be imparted.

THE NEGATIVE TRANSFERENCE.

The negative transference may range from a mild dislike to an intense and violent hate and loathing. Even a moderate degree impedes the analysis which cannot proceed easily in a hostile atmosphere. Like the

[1] Resistance, see p. 99.

G

positive form, it needs watching, and the same two sources of information are to be utilised. Unpunctuality, telephoning at the last moment to cancel the apointment, failing to attend at all, making outside appointments which clash with the hour, going away on a holiday, breaking off the treatment altogether —these are some of the evidences of the negative phase. Comments on your uncomfortable couch, queer taste in pictures, inattentive hall-maid, and so on, may be expected. The dreams similarly give expression to the negative feeling, and the analyst now finds himself identified with objects of the patient's dislike or contempt— a charwoman, farm-labourer or other menial, a boiler-cleaner or stoker ; a pig, a mule, and so on. In one of my cases the patient, during a negative phase, summed up her opinion of the analyst by dreaming of him as the village idiot.

Among other effects of a negative transference on the patient's behaviour, mention may be made of the following :—obstructing the analysis in order that the case may be a failure and so to the discredit of the physician ; pertinaciously attempting to make him lose his temper, and thereby prove himself no better than his patient ; bringing false charges and imputing wrong motives ; complaints of his behaviour, especially bullying, arrogance, want of sympathy or intelligence; mistrust and suspicion ; and, among medical patients, rejection of a psychological causation of their symptoms in favour of an organic diagnosis.

A remarkable effect of too strong a transference (and this applies equally to the positive form) is that first recognised by Freud,[1] namely, that the patient ceases to be able to recall memories, and instead merely reacts to the present situation in the same way as to the original one. This, perhaps, needs a word by way of elucidation. Suppose some feature in the patient's current behaviour is to be taken up for analysis—let us say, to quote a case, intense annoyance and dejection lasting many hours after a fellow-railway passenger had shown some unwillingness to lend his morning newspaper. Under other conditions of the transference the patient would recall

---

[1] *Internat. Zeitsch. f. Aertz. Psycho-analyse*, I., 2.

earlier and earlier incidents when he responded in this way to real or imagined thwarting, and would finally reach the childhood occasions when he first displayed this peculiarity. But when the transference is strong, none of these memories is accessible, and the analyst, in trying to help find them, will merely provoke the same intense annoyance and dejection in respect of himself. This kind of response, of course, blocks all further progress until the transference has been reduced.

In the earlier stages of the analysis it is, as a rule, useless to attempt to deal with negative manifestations straight away ; they are better left until the patient has become less negative. But in the later stages he will be ready to recognise them at once for what they are. In face of any such negative expression the physician's course is plain : he never allows his own negative feelings to be provoked, nor is he in the least hurt or intimidated. Equally necessary is it for him to abstain from going out of his way to conciliate his patient ; this could not fail to give the impression that he is running after him, and is anxious to soothe him—in other words, that the patient, by showing temper, can obtain some hold over him. On the contrary, as the patient becomes negative so the physician withdraws from him. He becomes more distant, leaving him to come back of his own accord. Nevertheless, he holds himself always ready to respond to any positive indication, and this is usually the moment when the negative phase can most usefully be analysed.

An interesting difference between the possible effects of positive and negative transference must be pointed out. Positive transference provides the patient with no motive for breaking off the treatment, which, other circumstances allowing, will be continued to its completion. But a strong negative transference urges him to break off the analysis forthwith. It is no uncommon thing to be told, as a patient is leaving, that he is not coming any more ; but cooler counsels usually prevail. With some, however, this hostility mounts to such a height that they break away altogether—one such patient telephoned that he could not bear the thought of even seeing me again. Now when an analysis has been completed, the patient soon ceases to be

interested in the physician, and forgets him.
After an incomplete analysis brought to an
end by external causes and during a positive
phase, the patient is likely to carry away and
spread an unduly favourable opinion of the
physician ; but these cases, as already mentioned, are necessarily few.   When, however,
the analysis is terminated on account of
negative transference, the patient is likely to
carry away and spread an unduly bad report ;
and these cases are much commoner.   It is
an adverse risk inseparable from analytical
work.

Since transference of either kind is an
obstacle and may, if it becomes strong, be
fatal to the treatment, we must know how to
deal with it and " dissolve " it.   Here pre-
vention is better than cure, and the first
need is to keep a close watch as it grows day
by day.   For the time being no active interference is called for, but so soon as it is evident
that it has reached the point of becoming an
impediment it must be taken in hand.   To
allow it to pass unrecognised or to grow to
large proportions is a serious mistake which

may take long to rectify. Here we come upon one of the most difficult practical tasks of all. To confront the patient bluntly with the fact would be worse than useless. In a positive case almost certain denial and a sense of injury, if not an equivalent negative change, would follow ; in a negative case an even more emphatic denial and an intensified negative feeling would result. We need to have at our disposal all the facts proving the existence of the transference—not only those we have observed ourselves but more especially those furnished by the patient in his associations— and placing these before him, to get him to draw his own conclusion. For this purpose a dream may be invaluable and often provides the clearest and most convincing testimony. Sooner or later, and generally sooner, a dream is brought in which the physician appears, however disguised, and, as already mentioned, the associations to the thought of this figure will include the patient's feelings and motives towards him at the moment. As soon as he recognises the identity of the figure (and this rarely presents any difficulty) he will usually acknowledge with conviction that the associations he has just given are his intimate thoughts about the analyst.

This, however, is only the first step. The transference is admitted by the patient, but it is not thereby dissolved. The next is to take up and analyse whatever motive has declared itself in the dream—affection, spite, jealousy, and so on—in order to trace its genesis (perhaps some trivial happening within the past few days, and this will itself link up with earlier occasions) and the advantage the patient wishes to gain by it. This insight is usually enough to dissolve the feeling at any rate temporarily, though the analyst will now be prepared for its return at any time, and can then deal with it at once as it has already been recognised by the patient.

After a few such instances the patient has experience enough to allow of some generalisation, and to begin to understand the nature and conditions of his own transference. It will be possible for him to see *from his own case* how his feelings for the analyst have varied from time to time, and how each new phase has depended, not as he supposed on a change in the physician, but on the psychical material being dealt with at the time. In this way he begins to grasp the nature of the transference, and recognises that the analyst has not provoked the feelings, but serves merely as a receptacle for them after their unrepression from the unconscious. This places him in a position to withdraw them and keep them henceforth at his own disposal.

This marks the second stage in the fate of the transference. In the first, the emotional repressions which have deprived the patient of the full vigour of his character are broken down, and the liberated energy is directed to the analyst as transference—a temporary arrangement, a half-way house as we have spoken of it. In the next this transference is dissolved, and the patient comes into free possession of all his impulses ; for the time being, and for want of useful outlets for them, this is likely to be a period of unrest and dissatisfaction. But in the third and last stage, which synchronises with the later months of the analysis and extends for months or years afterwards, he is finding for himself the objects in the attainment of which he intends to employ this new-found energy.

It is very necessary that even at this last stage the responsibility should be left with the patient. It is for him to choose and to decide. Only to this extent is the physician to intervene, namely, to indicate from his experience the various directions in which the happiest outlets are usually to be found. His advice will be in general terms rather than particular—as an everyday example, that a homosexual tendency finds its best outlet and sublimation in work on behalf of those of the same sex as the patient. But just how this is to be applied and translated into action must be left to the patient. However difficult this may seem to him at first, he can always rely on this assurance, that the whole force of natural development tends strongly towards health—in mental as in bodily disease, " Nature is on the side of the Physician."

The more difficult cases—those in which the solution of the transference is not effected as smoothly as has been represented above—will be those of patients who are capable of strong love or strong hate, and who are liable to be swept away by their feelings. The negative cases are pretty sure to bring the analysis to a vioent end themselves ; the positive may need to be ended, if necessary with some violence. With regard to the latter, the difficulty is not so great as might be supposed, especially if the analyst always bears in mind that as neurotics are sensitive and their craving for sympathy is limitless, he must allow for this in his handling of them. To be as gentle as possible is, after all, synonymous with being as firm as is necessary. Provided, therefore, he has been careful never to allow himself to provoke a patient's feelings, the necessary firmness in dealing with these strongly positive cases will rarely leave any ill-will behind. In the few cases where the patient is of a revengeful nature, this may not be avoidable, but no blame rests on the analyst. Indeed, he will find that no matter how scrupulously fair he may be, it is not possible to avoid unintentional hurts and their consequences. Some quite trivial remark or action on his part may call forth an emotional response

which takes weeks to subside. " Just one
rather less friendly remark," says Ferenczi,
" and the hate and rage of the patient will
follow " ; and, he might have added, that
just one word more friendly than usual may
call forth the liveliest fantasies of affection.

To bring this chapter to an end, let me give
a couple of illustrative cases. They are fairly
typical examples of strong transference, the
first negative, the other positive.

The patient in the first case was a professional man well in his thirties. The few ex-
planatory facts about him that need mention
are these. He was unmarried, and still lived
with his father. An only son, he early showed
himself possessed of overflowing physical
energy and a strong character which made
him but little disposed to submit to parental
authority, and which led him into innumerable breaches of paternal law. On the other
hand his father, who was middle-aged when
the boy was born, and even then was old-
fashioned, possessed a very hard, unaccom-
modating nature ; the obstinacy with which
he adhered to his views and ways of life was
a byword among his relatives, while as a

member of a strict religious sect he conceived it his duty to make his child conform in every way to the standards accepted by the elders of his church. With such a father such a son could develop only in one way ; the obstinacy in the boy grew as he had to defend himself against his father's stubbornness, and his dislike of him deepened into intense hate under the influence of incessant thwarting and punishment, including almost weekly thrashings. But as he came to adult years he recoiled from the thought of this hatred of his father, now old, widowed and almost friendless, and disposed of it by repression. The relations between them improved, " but then," my patient explained grimly, " I have taken master's place."

In the analysis his attitude to the physician was that to his father—a superficial friendliness thinly veiling hostility and antagonism. The greater part of the earlier work was occupied by his conflicts with his father, and the feelings thereby aroused soon led to the appearance of a negative transference. First he began to complain that I was unfair ; then that I always seemed to take the oppo-

site view to his own ; finally, that I was bent
on opposing him.   This negative transference
came to a sudden head one day when his
anger so seized him that he strode up and
down the room, shouting and shaking his fists,
and declaring that I was the biggest bully he
had ever met.   He had felt for several days
that I was laying myself out to quarrel, I
had provoked the quarrel that afternoon and
it was useless to go further with the analysis.
To this decision he adhered, and I never saw
him again.

As an example of positive transference, I
take the case of a patient who came, not with
anything approaching a neurosis, but because
she found life so miserable that she had
suicidal impulses which frightened her, and,
though possessing more than average intelligence, she was unable to maintain interest in
anything she applied herself to.   She was 23
and unmarried ; when she was quite a child
her mother, a neurotic, took to livng abroad
most of the year on the score of ill-health,
leaving the children to their father.   His
favourite among them was my patient, who
on her side developed little less than a blind

worship of him. In winter he usually came home after the other children were asleep, but this one was still awake, and he would sit on her bed till nearly dinner-time talking or even consulting her as though she were the mother. These half-hours when she had her father to herself were especially precious, and the memories of them were the tenderest she knew. The war, however, caused them to be separated ; they had not met since and correspondence was almost impossible.

Here again the attitude of the patient towards the physician was that towards her father—affection and trust. This enabled the analysis to go on a-pace, and though the positive transference gradually increased, the smoothness of the progress was never disturbed—until one morning it was apparent from her changed demeanour that the transference had suddenly flared up during the previous twenty-four hours. In the exaggeration of her dream of that night I was associated with Goethe, her literary hero, and with an emperor who is the largest figure in the history of his country. The following morning the associations came to a standstill, and, though deeply agitated, she spoke hardly a word. Later that morning, after leaving, she pencilled a note to me saying she felt she was going mad and could not wait for her appointment on the morrow; would I meet her at a certain concert that afternoon?

As I knew her to be shy to a degree and diffident where men were concerned, the unwonted courage she showed in writing in this way could only be further proof of the strength of the transference. But after reviewing every detail in the analysis of the past week or more in order to discover the cause of this sudden ebullition, I failed to find or even to suspect the occasion; nothing charged with any strong feeling had been brought up during these days. Admitting myself entirely at a loss, I awaited the appointment for the following day. She at once referred to the letter, and was covered with confusion as she apologised for it. The altered state of the transference was equally inexplicable to her, and we agreed to analyse the situation forthwith. The result is instructive.

In my room, at the foot of the couch, I

keep a rug, folded, for the use of any patient who may feel cold during the hour. In the present case the analysis was in the winter months, and for a week or more the weather had been bitterly cold, but my patient was too timid to avail herself properly of this cover ; instead she would first draw it over her ankles, then, as she got colder, to her knees, until in half-a-dozen moves she at last brought it nearly to her shoulders. I confess that this annoyed me, partly because each movement interrupted the associations and meant some loss of time in settling down again, and partly because I like people to go through with a thing once they begin, and not give up half way. However, I contented myself with letting her know that the rug was there expressly for use against the cold. But the next day the effect of this encouragement had passed off, and when she began the same hesitating movements again, I crossed from my chair to the couch, shook the rug open, and threw it over her from foot to neck.

As chance would have it, this was precisely what her father used to do in the winter-time when she was a child in bed and he

H

was saying good-night. Always as a last thing, he would take up the quilt and throw it over her just as I did the rug. In a moment my unconsidered action stirred a depth of tender memories, and it was from these that came the rush of feeling that seemed so unaccountable.

If further proof be needed of the correctness of this explanation, it is provided by the effect of the recognition of it on her part. The strength of the transference rapidly subsided ; within two or three days it was back at its old level, and the analysis was going ahead as before.

CHAPTER V

THE RESISTANCE

FROM whatever standpoint we may regard an analysis, its main purpose is to open up the patient's entire store of memories from earliest childhood onward. A proportion of these are, of course, available without any outside help, but the others, including many of the greatest importance, are so completely lost sight of and buried, that he could affirm with all honesty that they have no part in his mental life. Nevertheless it is often possible, as was mentioned previously, to infer for ourselves the existence of some unremembered memory, long before the patient has recalled it ; this we are able to do from observing his behaviour and the sentiments he expresses. We need not be in the least astonished at this apparent obliteration of even significant memories—under hypnosis events can readily be recalled of which no recollection exists in a waking state—and we must be prepared for denials which later have to be retracted.

These forgotten memories owe their repression to the painful affective tone which they possess. They may have been unpleasant from the first ; often they come to this by gradually establishing mental associations with some still earlier unpleasant memory ; but most frequently they were even intensely pleasant at the time, and only in retrospect when viewed in the light of a later cultural development, do they become charged with shame, remorse, and so on. Whichever way the repression began, the result is a blank—amnesia ; and as a rule, the more painful the memory the more powerful the repression directed against it. Analysis, then, aims at filling in all amnesiæ, and restoring the broken continuity from infancy onward. In the end the patient, having overcome his repressions and at the same time having freed his unconscious from the pent-up emotions associated with them, is able to review every stage and detail in his history without any emotional bias which would otherwise cloud his reason and warp his judgment in his present-day life.

Unlike any other kind of psycho-therapy, psycho-analysis is directed primarily and essentially against the repressions. But an act of repression is to be regarded dynamically as the exercise of so much psychical force. It can be overcome only by a counter-force of greater strength. Our next concern, therefore, is with this counter-force. Where is it to be found, and how employed? It comes in part from the patient and in part from the physician. A patient approaching a repression turns away from it so easily, naturally and unconsciously, as not to be in the least aware that his thoughts have glanced off at a tangent, and are receding from the very memory he is in need of finding. The physician, however, by indications which will be detailed immediately, recognises what is happening, and it is for him to bring the patient back to the path he has quitted. This may not be easy, and often is very difficult, but it is precisely on these occasions that he must be ready to put forth his own psychical energy to compel and hold his patient's attention to the repression. Incidentally, we have here the chief reason why analytical work is fatiguing to the physician. For be it noted that to overcome one repression by no means implies that all henceforth is smooth-going. On the contrary, each new represssion—and they are legion in every case—is retreated from as though no earlier one had been wrestled with. In other words, an analysis implies a continued battle with the patient, day after day and month after month. Indeed, it could not be otherwise, even in cases that are going most favourably, because as soon as one repression has been overcome, the next must be attacked.

All the time the patient will be opposing. His endeavour is to circumvent, retreat, escape, and these attempts can be countered only by the persistence of the analyst, who nevertheless cannot himself overcome the resistance. The most he can do when he has led the patient back to the repression, is to induce him to recognise that he is resisting. Only then is the patient in a position to bring into play his own counterforce, and by his own volition and determination to break through the repression. Once he has made up his mind to do this, the resistance disappears, the repression is overcome, and the memory emerges. All this implies considerable mental effort—much more than is claimed from the analyst—and few patients fail to comment on the exhausting effect of an hour's work.[1]

But supposing the physician should be one who has not overcome his resistances—shows, that is to say, counter-resistance—what sort of help can he be to his patient? With one as blind as the other, neither can see the resistance and both will turn unconsciously from it. " Just so far as the physician has got the better of his own repressions, so far are his services of value to his patients—but no farther." The full significance of this statement in Chapter I will now be apparent.

---

[1] If we were to seek a comparison that might make this contest clearer, I know of none better than trying to take an unwilling horse over a hurdle. The horse may come almost abreast of the jump, and then swerve and go off in another direction ; it may jib and refuse to approach it at all ; it may buck and try to throw its rider. It will sometimes stop dead this side of the hurdle and the rider goes over alone ; even this has its counterpart in the analysis where the technically inefficient analyst communicates to the patient the knowledge he is resisting, to find that the two have parted company, and that he has gone on, but his patient is still confronted by the resistance.

Since the responsibility of detecting resistances falls on the analyst, it is imperative he should know by what indications to recognise them. These signs are very numerous and for descriptive purposes may be placed in three groups—those expressing direct opposition to the analysis, as by refusing to conform to its conditions ; those in which the opposition is indirect, such as deceiving and misleading the physician ; those in which some special motive is indulged.

By far the commonest form of direct opposition is to set aside the injunction invariably given to " speak every thought that comes to your mind." Now it is a fact, never to be lost sight of, that with anyone who is given over to free association, the current of thought is unintermitting ; idea follows idea in quick succession, now a verbal memory, now a visual one, and so on, and the difficulty is to keep pace with the flow that brims the mind. Any check to it is the work of the resistance ; and the interruption that follows may be anything from a momentary hesitation to a protracted silence. In these longer periods the patient is pretty sure to explain that it is not a matter of a thought being withheld, but that his mind is a blank. He may then be reminded that free associations flow without intermission, and asked to accept, if only provisionally as a working hypothesis, the assurance that he is resisting some idea or train of ideas which is waiting to emerge. He is directed to give his attention, not at all to the missing memory, but to the nature of the resistance ; to carry his mind back to the point where the chain of associations broke, to pick up the thread where he lost it, and to say what thought or wave of feeling caused the interruption. This found, its significance is then dealt with by discussion, after which the resisted memory will come to hand readily enough. From the foregoing the beginner will understand that a direct attempt to find the resisted memory is technically wrong, the correct procedure being to concentrate on the resistance behind which the memory is hidden.

Most often this resistance will be found to involve some reference to the physician himself. In the negative phase of the transference the patient's feelings are in some considerable measure against furthering the analysis, and thereby helping his supposed antagonist, the physician ; in the positive phase he finds difficulty in making any admission which he thinks may lower him in the physician's esteem.   In the former case, it may be pointed out that the analysis is for his benefit ; if he cares to obstruct it the loss is his, and the analyst can in no way feel responsible.   In the positive case, the analysis again is for the good of the patient who presumably did not undertake it in order to make a favourable impression on the physician.   In either case, the opinion and feelings of the analyst are of small account compared with the purpose of the treatment, which is to afford the patient a complete self-knowledge of the true facts of his life.

On many occasions the resistance is only partial, and the patient is willing to speak his thought provided he can first protect himself by a preliminary statement transferring the responsibility for it to someone else.   It is especially common for a patient, on nearing the unpalatable conclusion of a chain of memories, to remark to the analyst, " I know what *you* are thinking," or " I know

what you want me to say "—and then comes
the resisted thought. In this way he endeavours to evade responsibility by fathering
the memory on to the analyst—it is he who
has put it in his mind ; it is his suggestion.
This, of course, is an example of the well-
known mechanism of " projection " of ideas ;
and the patient's attention may be drawn to
the fact.

Another form taken by the resistance is
that first mentioned by Freud, in which the
patient insists he has already spoken of
something which in fact he has not mentioned. What has happened is that the
thoughts have been in his mind and he has
had the intention of speaking them, but in the
event passed them over unspoken—in the
phraseology of a committee-book, they were
" taken as read." Unless, however, the
analyst is quite confident of his own memory,
he would do well on these occasions to be
ready to ascribe the forgetfulness to himself,
at any rate, until further evidence is forth-
coming.

Yet another expression of the resistance
must be mentioned, one which may be dis-

concerting to the student. I refer to those patients—usually with largely negative and narcissistic temperaments—who, whenever a resistance is approached, react by an outburst of anger and indignation against the physician. The latter, needless to say, does not respond to this in kind ; there is more likelihood of him being intimidated and retreating, leaving the patient master of the situation. But once he recognises the meaning of the outbursts, and that the patient is one of those whose habit it is to defend themselves against criticism by a show of aggression, he will know how to deal with him.

Of the more indirect ways in which the resistance shows itself, mention may be made of the following. Instead of acting as an obstacle to the flow of thought, it endeavours to gain its end by associations so profuse as to whelm and obscure the case. The patient talks incessantly, but keeps to the surface, and at the end of the hour has said little or nothing of any value towards disclosing the deeper levels of his mind. Long, prolix dreams are brought with unfailing regularity, but nothing emerges from their analysis.

These discursive associations were referred to in Chap. III (p. 50), where it was explained that the patient, when taxed with them, usually defends himself by insisting on the scrupulously thorough way in which he is obeying his instruction to speak every thought. When, later, it is pointed out to him that no real progress is being made, he cheerfully disclaims all responsibility ; he is doing what was asked of him, and the failure plainly lies with the method of psycho-analysis itself. To counter this, it may be well to explain that these superficial associations almost always represent an endeavour to evade an obstacle lying immediately ahead. Can this be so in his case ? What topic can he find near the surface of his thoughts which he is little willing to speak about ? In the case of lengthy dreams no attempt should be made to analyse more than a part, or to resume on the following day the analysis of what has been left over. The rule here, as always with dream-analysis, is to take each day the dream of the previous night, even though yesterday's dream has been left in-completely analysed. The importance of this lies in the need of keeping in close touch with the daily aspect of the unconscious—with its living surface.   Nothing will be lost in the long run by laying aside an incompleted dream analysis ; whatever part of it has not been dealt with will surely reappear again and again in subsequent dreams until at last it receives attention.

In other cases this veiled resistance takes other forms.   In some an apparent keen interest is shown in everything psycho-analytical.   The wish is expressed to " understand " it all "thoroughly," and detailed explanations are asked for at every point—but the analysis progresses not at all.   In others, a considerable portion of the hour is consumed in recounting the happenings since the visit of the day before.   In others again, the endeavour is made to keep things on the plane of an ordinary conversation into which the analyst is to be drawn by directly asking his views and opinions.

Rather more difficult cases are those in which a natural obstinacy is invoked in support of the resistance.   This shows itself in two ways particularly.   In the one an apparent readiness to accept and acquiesce in everything, masks an underlying determination to yield not an inch ; " If you say so, of course it is so," sums up this attitude to the physician. In the other the obstinacy is responsible for what is nothing but assumed stupidity. Each time the patient is asked to face a resistance he declares he doesn't understand, he can't follow you, he doesn't know what you mean ; but at all other times he is quick enough. A special form of this is sometimes seen when as a last prevarication before taking the plunge, the plea is put forward that, although the resisted memory is now recognised, the correct words in which to express it are not available ; this excuse is most frequent in the intelligent and well-educated who at no other time find need to asperse their vocabularies.

So far we have been speaking only of the resistance as it shows itself at each fresh step. It is most often connected with feelings of shame which make it hard for the patient to bring himself to face the successive inscriptions on the record of his past ; this difficulty is, of course, all the greater if he is of a narcissistic disposition. We have now to recognise some additional resistances, even deeper and more widespread, which come to be directed not so much against each successive advance as against the treatment as a whole. Here we light upon motives, some of them common, but others present in by no means all patients, which, until they are got out of the way—and this is generally difficult, and sometimes impossible—put a successful ending out of the question.

First among them must be named the wish not to get well, the wish to retain the neurosis. This is very common, if only because almost every neurotic has learned to turn his nervous disabilities to his own advantage, and he is, therefore, to a greater or less extent reluctant to part with them. Whether it be merely a nervous headache which has become a convenient excuse for avoiding irksome duties and social calls, or whether it be a matter of a paralysis which confines the patient to bed, whence the household can be dominated by this mute appeal to sympathy, a neurotic trouble lends itself very readily to use in these directions ; and, of course, as long as a neutoric wishes not to be cured, there is no curing him. In an analysis this motive needs to be identified early, but before this can be done the physician must have all the necessary proof provided by his patient before he can piece it together in such a way as to bring conviction. Once this has been done, however, he need waste no time in pointing to it whenever it shows subsequently. A special expression of this motive is that in which a patient tries to prolong the treatment (even to his personal cost) in order to prove his case incurable.

Another motive met with more often than might be supposed is spite against the analyst. Here the wish is to prove a failure in order to disappoint him and damage his reputation. It is, of course, a negative sadistic type of patient who indulges this impulse, but usually there is no great difficulty in clearing it out of the way.

Quite otherwise, however, is that special combination of negative and narcissistic traits which is responsible for a type of patient who is convinced he knows everything better than the analyst, and would take the entire treatment into his own hands. This disposition shows itself, as Abraham points out,[1] in a full measure of opposition to the physician, a strong disinclination to submit to his directions, and a wish, into which envy enters, to prove himself the better man. The ambivalent attitude to the father is well seen here —rejection of his claims to superiority, and at the same time the wish to possess and exercise his qualities. Interestingly enough, patients of this type rarely break off the analysis, but are willing to continue it for many months, so great is the satisfaction they find in conducting the treatment themselves.

Among other types presenting special difficulty reference must be made to the following :—The masochistic : in these the masochistic tendency is responsible for an unhappy pleasure in misfortunes. In their every-day life they take a secret delight in seeing their plans go wrong and their hopes frustrated ; they feel real enjoyment in being unfairly used, victimised and martyred ; and they will often, though quite unconsciously, so engineer things as to bring trouble upon

[1] *Internat. Zeitschrift für Psycho-analyse*, vol. V., p. 173.

themselves. To these the sufferings and disabilities of a neurosis are very sweet, and it
need hardly be said that they are among the
more difficult subjects for analysis. In
another type of patient suspiciousness is a
leading trait, and the physician finds his
every word and effort misinterpreted in a
hostile atmosphere. The patient is entirely
unable to repose any trust in him, or to
believe that any good can come of the treatment. If, as is often the case, this mistrust
is linked with paranoic characters, a particularly unfavourable subject is the result.
Yet another type is the patient, usually with
an outstanding neurosis since early school-
days, who, on this account, was petted and
spoiled as a child and since, and is too selfish
and lacking in moral fibre to take any but the
line of least resistance. To find that the
analysis is an appeal to his attenuated sense
of responsibility may be more than he can
tolerate.

To complete this brief enumeration, we
should just mention those in whom deceit
and lying are ingrained traits ; those with
excessive narcissism ; those of shallow nature,

with few principles other than that of expediency, and neither the wish nor the ability to sublimate their impulses ; and, finally, the very stubborn.

Not that any in this list, except the penultimate, is beyond the reach of psychoanalysis, but all of them present special difficulties, and for this reason slower progress and longer treatment is to be expected. When, however, several of these obstacles are combined in one and the same patient, the problem is all the harder, and if many of them go together the hope of any substantial success is correspondingly small. These cases, however, are exceptional.

From what has been said in the foregoing pages, the reader will understand that the resistance is one of the larger factors on which success depends. Yet it is a factor which in the present state of analytical knowledge cannot be gauged except by actual trial in each patient. At the outset of a case it is largely an unknown factor, and to this extent the result of the treatment must be doubtful. Neither the strength of the resistance nor the patient's ability to overcome it can be foreseen ; and, in particular, the more powerful motives come to light only as the analysis proceeds. With these latter it is not to be supposed that every patient will prove resolute in mastering them, notwithstanding the harm they do him. Sometimes the struggle will swing this way and that for weeks or months, to end in definite failure or definite success. We can only watch it, and help as opportunity offers ; but more often than not it ends in success. Let this be remembered in those toilsome cases where the fight goes on and on day after day, and the patient seems to lack the strength of mind to give up the advantages his neurosis gains for him, to strip away the narcissism which blinds him to the true facts of his illness, or to renounce the masochistic desire to cherish his misfortunes. Even though his good intentions and ability may seem almost hopeless, the current may set in any day in the right direction, and within a short time he begins to free himself from some of his most serious failings.

Perhaps, in looking for a case that will help to make clearer some of the chief points in this chapter, I shall do best to choose a difficult one, even though it is out of the ordinary. The following case—to be described only so far as the resistance is concerned—with its combination of a number of adverse features, was exceptionally hard to deal with, and went no further than a partial improvement.

Before coming to me the patient, a business man nearing middle-age, intelligent and well-read, had for several years been under treatment of some kind or other, including ordinary medical treatment, sea-voyages, hydropathic treatment, Christian science, suggestion, and at least two courses of analysis. Nevertheless he embarked on a third with unexpected hopefulness, and at once made arrangements to continue it for several months. Throughout the whole time he was amiable, never missed or was late for his appointment, and for a while associated freely. He rarely failed to bring a dream, and even kept pencil and paper at his bedside to use in the middle of the night or immediately after waking. In fact, the way he persisted in doing this after having been told it was unnecessary, gave the first hint of what was amiss with him. Gradually it became apparent that very slow progress was being made, his associations rarely went outside the ground covered by his previous analysis, and every attempt to bring him back to a resistance led only to a further repetition of old associations. He recognised we were not making headway, but said he felt sure from the outset that there was something wrong in my technique ; in proof thereof he quoted various works on psycho-analysis. To my recommendation not to read these books but to learn from his own case, he responded by continuing to obtain and read all new books that appeared. He became more openly critical of me, readier in suggesting how the analysis should be made, and finally claimed to know more of the subject than I did.

It was evident that (intellectual) narcissism was a strong component of his character and would prove a serious hindrance in the analysis. In spite of this, however, some little progress was made, but whenever enough fresh material had been obtained to give some

further insight into his illness, the reply was
" I quite understand all that, but what's the
good ?   Understanding isn't going to make
me any better." Yet on other occasions his
complaint was that as I did not seem to try
to make him understand, how could he possibly get better ?   Either way he was not
going to let himself get better.   Here then
was one of those cases with a motive for remaining ill.   What, then, did he stand to lose
if he got well ?   He was a partner in a business founded by his father (a strong and
capable business man), into which he had
been taken much against his will on leaving
school.   The character of the work and
business life itself were distasteful to him, and
he could never forgive his father for forcing
him into it.   He had never ceased to want to
get out again, but it was only the increasing
severity of his neurosis which had at last,
after many years, obtained for him a long
leave of absence.   But if he recovered——.

The father, however, had been dead many
years.   And yet the patient had never been
able to bring himself to resign, although his
financial interest was safeguarded.   The ex-

planation of this irresolution was that his father would not have approved of him leaving, and he still felt he could not go against his wishes. His childhood memories confirmed this, and showed the strong ambivalency of his feelings towards his father. He had a great admiration for him with his quiet, successful personality. But he was the youngest child, born after an interval of many years—in point of fact, an " accident " —and unwanted by his father, who was already getting old and had neither time nor affection to spare for any child. Quite early the boy was told that his father did not want him ; for this he hated him, and inevitably this hate generated fear. The years of his childhood had been dominated by this curious dual influence of his father—love and admiration for him, and the resolve to make him his perfect pattern of manhood ; fear, hate and rebellion, and the determination to break away from every standard his father upheld. Even now, as a man, he showed the same domination—the strongest never-ceasing impulses to offend every convention, but the keenest remorse whenever he fell below the level set by his conscience ; as a patient, the most amicable feelings for the analyst, but a determination to submit to him in no way.

The wish not to get well was powerfully reinforced from two other directions. He foresaw that his anti-social proclivities would not survive a successful analysis, and he had no inclination to bring this side under control. Further, his neurosis had obtained for him special consideration and forbearance from his boyhood onward—especially from his mother and later from his wife. There had always been others to shoulder his responsibilities ; he realised that to part with his neurosis would mean self-dependence, and from this he shrank. "I don't really want to get well," was his summary of the position.

These motives for resistance should have have been enough for one case, but there were others to come. The masochistic tendency was strong, and he was conscious of the keenest pleasure when people commiserated him. Why, therefore, deprive himself of the ground that drew their sympathy ? His policy in life was to offer the other cheek to the smiter ; another guiding principle, adopted as a boy, was that if he could not get what he wanted he would make himself a martyr.

Yet again he was extremely suspicious by nature, and mistrusted literally everything I said. It was a duty, he said, to mistrust everyone. In keeping with this he was conscious of seeking to deceive himself as well as others. " Pretending without intending " and " Ostensibly to conform, really to evade " were two more of his aphorisms of life ; and they guided him at most points in the treatment. Lying and hypocrisy were motives which often appeared in his dreams, and indeed his dream-symbol of himself was a fox—" a clever, cunning, treacherous animal." To be mentally honest, he once declared, one must throw one's weight on one side or the other, and this he never could do. The ambivalency which was so marked a feature of the case not only prevented him from knowing his own mind on any subject, but interfered with almost every action—" Whenever I feel an urge to do anything," he once said, " at once comes an inhibition." Finally, as might be supposed, obstinacy played a large part in his behaviour, and constantly sought its end in the analytical work by deliberate opposition, by assured stupidity, and by a pretence of agreeing.

A personality which included all these features could not be other than exceptionally difficult for analytical purposes, and needed correspondingly prolonged treatment. In the present case, however, it terminated abruptly and characteristically after several months. The patient stayed away for two days. On his return he reported that he had resigned from his business. The next day he said he felt he could get no without further treatment, and the analysis ended. From this it will be seen that he had at last succeeded in coming to grips with his father-complex, and after twenty years took his own course in life. This represents no small achievement. Though much remained to be put right, he had at any rate burst one of the bonds which restrained his development, and this should give room for new expansion.

CHAPTER VI

THE TERMINATION OF THE ANALYSIS

PATIENTS often come with the idea that in analytical cases it will be possible on a given day to tell them, " To-day everything has healed ; to-morrow go home." Or they suppose that once some particular memory is recovered, nothing more will be needed and all will be well with them. Unfounded as these notions are—since every neurosis is of gradual development and can only gradually be remedied—the choice of the best time for bringing the treatment to an end may be one of considerable difficulty, apart from external causes such as expense, business claims, persuasion of relatives, and the like.

In the first place an analysis which stops short of completely filling infantile amnesiæ may nevertheless be beneficial. Should it have gone no further than to apprise the patient of some of the unconscious forces chiefly responsible for his troubles in life, a restricted analysis is valuable. The ground recovered is never likely to be lost, and even more important, the healing process set in operation by releasing some of the repressions tends towards further recovery. Physician and patient alike may therefore be content even when more could be done had circumstances allowed.

But it is when no external cause need be taken into account that doubt may arise. In these cases the criterion is the fitness of the patient to meet the demands of everyday life. This is a matter on which judgment can be formed more easily than might be supposed. Throughout the earlier months the aim is to identify the unconscious material— complexes, fixations, repressed desires and impulses. In the later months this hard-won knowledge is to be applied to the patient's daily life. At this later stage the analyst, who has so far been a listener, moves into the foreground. Each day the patient brings an account of his difficulties during the past twenty-four hours—worries, irritabilities, moods, embarrassments—and it will be found that in spite of the work already done, he still tends by force of long habit to react to situations in much the same way as before. But the position is now fundamentally altered for the better, in that he is able, with the physician's help, rapidly to find the causes affecting his behaviour on each occasion. By keeping these in mind on the next and subsequent occasions when the same difficulty has to be faced, he pretty soon gains the self-control he wants, and before long finds himself facing the same situation not only without difficulty, but without realising till afterwards that he has accomplished without a thought what hitherto has meant nervous strain and failure.

Hand in hand with this goes the gradual sublimation of the liberated energy now at his disposal. This process is likely to continue long after the treatment is over. Meanwhile the physician should bear two considerations in mind. The amount and degree of sublimation that is possible varies from one case to another, and to set too high a standard is injurious. That standard is best which is the highest compatible with both mental and physical health. The second consideration—it was mentioned in an earlier chapter—is that the patient is to be given the same freedom and independence in choosing the manner and extent of his sublimations as is urged upon him by psycho-analysis in all his decisions. To advise, except in general terms, and still worse, to press suggestions, is no part of the analyst's function ; if this position is departed from, unsuccessful experiments and disappointment on both sides will result. Indeed, the physician, as an interested onlooker, will sometimes have occasion to reflect, when his patient follows a course which is not the one he himself had in mind as best, that the patient's choice proves wisest in the event. In other words, what seems and is best for one, may be second or third best for another.

It is, however, the duty of the physician persistently to keep in the patient's full view all the impulses which have been made conscious ; this is needed to counteract the almost invariable tendency to forget. By daily paradigms, as it were, the patient learns the healthy control and utilisation of these impulses, and with increasing practice becomes more apt until, instead of bringing several or a few or one difficulty during the previous twenty-four hours, he comes one day with nothing on which he needs help. Now is the time to cut down his attendances —every second day, twice a week, weekly, will be often enough.   In this way almost the last threads of the transference will break ; he ceases even to wish to rely on the analyst or anyone else, and henceforth is self-dependent. This is the goal the physician has aimed at from the beginning.   His parting advice to his patient will be in most cases to trouble himself no more with psycho-analysis or with psycho-analysts, but to make the best of life and enjoy it.   To the more intelligent moiety of them he will add the recommendation to keep themselves in touch with the unconscious by analysing their own dreams.

Not always, however, will the ending be this smooth.   The exceptions are likely to be the cases referred to on an earlier page in which the transference, positive or negative, is out of the ordinary.   A strong positive transference may come to be a leading motive for prolonging the treatment.   In such cases

K

it will generally be possible to dissolve it on the lines already indicated. Only very occasionally will this fail, but it is precisely in these cases that a forcible ending must not be shunned. Stekel, discussing the terminations of psycho-analytical treatments, inclines to the view that some cases must end with some degree of violence, and there can be no doubt that with patients in which the ability to sublimate is little developed, this termination is the best in the long run.

The difficulty with very negative cases lies rather in the other direction. The violent ending is to be expected, as has been already explained, rather from the patient than from any other source. Difficulty so far as the physician is concerned is more likely to arise where a strongly negative patient, as sometimes happens, is far from showing any disposition to break away, and yet weeks pass by with little or no progress. Should he advise the termination of the treatment in these circumstances ? The question is not easy to answer unequivocally, but in general it may be said that the circumstances do not justify this action. The reason for this is a practical one. Experience shows that in such cases, even when progress has long been held up and the analyst has almost abandoned hope of anything better, the day comes when the negative phase passes and satisfactory conditions are established.

Negative patients will sometimes ask, should they not seek some other analyst against whom they feel no personal dislike? If they do this the probability, from the very nature of their negative feeling, is that before long they will be as hostile to their new as they are to their first analyst. All the same, in some special cases I should incline to another view, since the change to an analyst of the other sex may be all to the good. Male patients, for example, who are strongly negative to the father (such as the case described on p. 92) may do better with a woman analyst ; the converse would hold of a female patient, negative to the mother. I would also mention as a special type in this connection, female patients with a strong castration-complex ; with these their jealousy of men and antagonism to them are fertile sources of analytical difficulties which would not be

likely to arise with a woman analyst. Nevertheless in all these cases the decision is not so
simple, because while, on the one hand, difficulties encountered by a man-analyst may
be of small consequence with a woman-
analyst, other difficulties might spring up
after the change which had been of no importance before. A further consideration
might be added. Healthy temperaments are
hostile to neither men nor women, and the
negatively disposed patient cannot be accounted normal until this hostility has passed
away. On the principle, therefore, that a
patient is not to be shielded from the irritant
causes of his neurosis there is ground for continuing even in face of strong negative
feeling. Nevertheless the treatment might be
shorter at the hands of another analyst, but
proof of this, of course, can never be forth-
coming.

For a last word let us epitomise in the
shortest possible form the subject which has
been presented in the foregoing chapters.

   1. Psycho-analytical treatment has for its
aim the opening up of infantile amnesiæ and

the restoring to consciousness of all childhood memories.

2. This work is obstructed by the resistance which prevents the return of these memories and keeps them represesd and unconscious. It is the resistance, therefore, that claims chief attention throughout.

3. To help in overcoming the resistance the positive transference is utilised. This transference is the sole warrant of the physician's authority. With its aid he enables recollections to be faced which would otherwise be too painful, and emotions to be liberated which have been repressed along with the memories.

4. In the result this pent-up emotional energy which alone is the source of neurotic symptoms, is released and, as a new flow of energy along consciously directed channels, brings added force and efficiency of character with which to meet the demands of social life.